Cholangiography After Orthotopic Liver Transplantation

Springer

Berlin
Heidelberg
New York
Barcelona
Budapest
Hong Kong
London
Milan
Paris
Santa Clara
Singapore
Tokyo

G. Nöldge · G. Otto · L. Theilmann

Cholangiography After Orthotopic Liver Transplantation

With 67 Figures

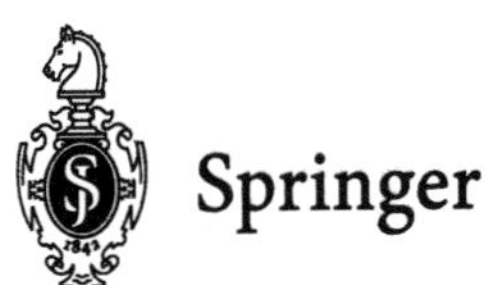

Springer

Prof. Dr. Gerd Nöldge
Department of Radiology
University of Heidelberg
Im Neuenheimer Feld 110
69120 Heidelberg
Germany

Prof. Dr. Gerd Otto
Department of Surgery
University of Heidelberg
Im Neuenheimer Feld 110
69120 Heidelberg
Germany

Prof. Dr. Lorenz Theilmann
Department of Internal Medicine
University of Heidelberg
Bergheimer Straße 58
69115 Heidelberg
Germany

ISBN-13: 978-3-540-60491-4   e-ISBN-13: 978-3-642-61064-6
DOI: 10.1007/978-3-642-61064-6

Cataloging-in-Publication Data applied for
Die Deutsche Bibliothek – CIP-Einheitsaufnahme
Nöldge, Gerd:
Cholangiography after orthotopic liver transplantation / G. Nöldge; G. Otto; L. Theil-
mann. – Berlin; Heidelberg; New York; Barcelona; Budapest; Hong Kong; London; Milan;
Paris; Santa Clara; Singapore; Tokyo: Springer, 1996
    ISBN-13: 978-3-540-60491-4
NE: Otto, Gerd; Theilmann, Lorenz:

Typesetting: K+V Fotosatz GmbH, Beerfelden
Reproduction of the figures: Schneider Repro GmbH, Heidelberg
Printing and binding: Graphischer Betrieb Konrad Triltsch, Würzburg

SPIN: 10521325   21/3135 - 5 4 3 2 1 0 – Printed on acid-free paper

Publication of this book was made possible by generous
support from the following companies:

Sandoz AG
Biotest Pharma GmbH
Immuno GmbH
Fujisawa GmbH
Boston Scientific GmbH
DuPont Pharma GmbH
Glaxo Wellcome GmbH
MSD Sharp & Dohme GmbH

Preface

Several years ago biliary tract reconstruction was regarded as the Achilles' heel of liver transplantation. Even though many technical improvements have been introduced into clinical practice, biliary tract complications have remained a cause of major morbidity and even of mortality.

The prognosis following liver transplantation may adversely be affected by numerous potential problems, such as reinfection of the graft, recurrence of primary hepatic disease, or chronic rejection, all of which are still uncorrectable. The majority of biliary complications can be avoided by appropriate surgical technique. In the case of manifest complications, experience in interventional radiology and endoscopy is essential in order to alleviate morbidity and to minimize the potential necessity of hospitalization or even surgery. The features and complexity of these diagnostic and therapeutic procedures have extraordinarily stimulated the cooperation between endoscopists, radiologists, and surgeons. This book reflects this intense clinical teamwork.

The titles of the following chapters do not strictly follow the radiological features or pathogenesis of bile duct alterations, but rather the clinical and therapeutic aspects which may be encountered in the early and late phases following liver transplantation in adults. The figures reproduced in this publication have been gathered from a review of cholangiograms from more than 200 patients who had undergone orthotopic liver transplantations. The purpose of this review was to draw on our personal experience and the generally accepted knowledge in order to provide a survey of the etiology, clinical aspects, and appropriate treatment of complications of clinical liver transplantation.

The authors would like to thank Prof. A. Stiehl from the Department of Gastroenterology, who was involved in the endoscopic procedures, for helpful discussions, Dr. T. Roeren from the Department of Radiology for performing percutaneous

biliary drainage, and Prof. G.W. Kauffmann, Chairman of the
Department of Radiology, for his continuous support. This
work is based on actual clinical liver transplantations, a procedure which was initiated in Heidelberg and continuously pro-
moted by Prof. C. Herfarth, Director of the Department of
General Surgery.

G. Nöldge
G. Otto
L. Theilmann

Contents

Bile Duct Stenosis Due to Local Ischemia

Ischemic-Type Lesions Following Long Cold Ischemia

Bile Duct Alterations After Occlusion of the Hepatic Artery

Bile Ducts in Chronic Rejection

Disturbed Function of the Sphincter of Oddi

Abbreviations

OLT   Orthotopic liver transplantation

ERC   Endoscopic retrograde cholangiography

ERCP   Endoscopic retrograde cholangio-pancreatico-
       graphy

Introduction: Biliary Reconstruction and Biliary Complications
Normal Cholangiogram Following Orthotopic Liver Transplantation

Short Overview

The surgical techniques most frequently used for biliary reconstruction are end-to-end choledocho-choledochostomy over a T-tube, choledocho-jejunostomy to a Roux-en-Y loop and, especially in Germany, side-to-side choledocho-choledochostomy [1, 8, 14, 21]. Techniques employed in the early years of liver transplantation, e.g., cholecysto-enterostomy of the gallbladder conduit (Waddell-Calne), have now been generally abandoned. We have used end-to-end and side-to-side choledocho-choledochostomy as well as biliodigestive reconstruction with similar results [29]. The technique we currently prefer is side-to-side anastomosis.

As a result of better anatomical understanding of the vascular supply of the biliary system and of improved surgical techniques for both biliary and arterial reconstruction, there has been progress in improving the outcome of biliary duct reconstruction. Any extended dissection of the bile duct of the graft should be avoided during surgery in order to preserve the integrity of periductal vessels; electrocauterization should not be used for the same reason. The blood supply to the bile duct usually stems from the gastroduodenal and right hepatic arteries, which are connected by three small arteries running along the bile duct [24, 32]. Since the connection to the right hepatic artery may be rather sparse, it can be impaired during surgery. The blood supply to the central portion of the left hepatic duct is also from the right hepatic artery. This is of importance in segmental (segments 2 and 3) and especially in split liver transplantation [28]. Despite the awareness of these anatomical features, biliary tract complications continue to occur more frequently after pediatric liver transplantation than after transplantation in adults [11]. In general, the causes of biliary tract complications are surgical technique, local ischemia, arterial occlusion, rejection of the graft, and the preservation solution. The lack of normal innervation of the bile ducts within but also outside the graft may lead to impaired motility and, thus, to ascending cholangitis which may be superimposed on preexisting minor abnormalities.

In the past biliary tract complications following orthotopic liver transplantation were reported to occur in 20%–40% of the cases [8, 13, 14, 37]. More recently, complication rates amount to 10%–20% [1, 7, 20, 29] (table). The main complications are bile duct stenoses, leakage and formation of casts or sludge in the biliary tree.

Clinical and radiological features do not correlate with particular causative factors. Arterial occlusion, for example, may result in a single stenosis, multiple strictures, leakage of the bile duct, or even sludge formation. The diagnostic and interventional approaches used in biliary complications following liver transplantation are identical to general techniques. Usually the biliary tree is first visualized through the T-tube or a small catheter which has been introduced via the cystic duct of the graft. After removal of these catheters, ERC or PTC are required. Interventional techniques include sphincterotomy by ERC, rinsing of the bile ducts, balloon dilation, and placement of prostheses or stents by both ERC and PTC.

Biliary Tract Complications after Liver Transplantation.
[a] References in [20], [b] related to biliary complications, [c] pediatric liver transplantation; C-C, choledocho-choledochostomy; C-RY, choledocho-jejunostomy; e-e, end-to-end; s-s, side-to-side

Author/ year/ reference	Type of anasto-mosis	Complication		Leakage (%)	Stenosis/ obstruc-tion (%)
		n	Total complication rate (%)		
Chaib 1994 [1]	All types of recon-struction	187	14	3.2	9.0
Greif 1994 [7]	All types of recon-struction	1792	11.5	3.2	5.2
	C-C	–	–	27.1[b]	36.4[b]
	C-RY	–	–	25.9[b]	52.9[b]
Hiatt 1987[a]	C-C	51	28	–	–
	C-RY	27	30	–	–
Lallier 1993 [11][c]	C-C	24	25	13.2	9.4
	C-RY	29	24		
Lerut 1987 [14]	C-C	159	12.6	–	–
	C-RY	175	5.2	–	–
Neuhaus 1994 [20]	C-C (s-s)	300	11.5	0.3	0.6
	C-RY	40			
Ringe 1989[a]	C-C (s-s)	156	8.5	3.8	0.6
	C-C (e-e)	41	35.9	17	2.4
	C-RY	84	23.8	11.9	2.4
Rouch 1990 [25]	C-C (wo. T-tube)	38	18	2.6	15.8
	C-C	26	35	19.2	7.7
	C-RY	72	21	12.5	6.9

Case 1 Normal Postoperative Cholangiogram Following OLT

History

A 51-year-old male patient underwent liver transplantation because of end-stage liver cirrhosis due to chronic hepatitis B virus infection. A routine cholangiogram was performed 2 weeks after orthotopic liver transplantation (OLT) (Fig. 1).

Cholangiogram

The intra- and extrahepatic biliary tract is visualized using a small-caliber catheter which has been inserted through the remnant cystic duct of the donor liver. The intra- and extrahepatic bile ducts are of normal size with a regular end-to-end choledochocholedochostomy without signs of leakage. There is quick flow of the contrast medium via the papilla into the duodenum. (A large drain caliber is still in place in the right upper quadrant.)

Case 2 Normal Postoperative Cholangiogram with a Certain Degree of Mismatch Between Common Bile Ducts of Donor and Recipient

History

A 23-year-old female patient received a liver graft because of liver cirrhosis due to chronic hepatitis C virus (HCV) infection. Endoscopic retrograde cholangiography (ERC) was performed 1 month after OLT because of an increase in the liver enzymes and bilirubin. Liver histology and detection of HCV RNA in serum revealed viral hepatitis due to recurrence of the hepatitis C virus infection.

Endoscopic Retrograde Cholangiopancreaticography (ERCP)

Normal cholangiogram after liver transplantation (Fig. 2). As usual, the donor's gall bladder has been removed. The donor's cystic duct is visualized as a 1-cm-long stump (*arrow*). A side-to-side choledochocholedochostomy has been performed. There is a slight mismatch between the diameters of the common bile ducts of donor and recipient. There is satisfactory bile flow via the papilla into the duodenum. The pancreatic duct in the head of the pancreas is weakly visualized.

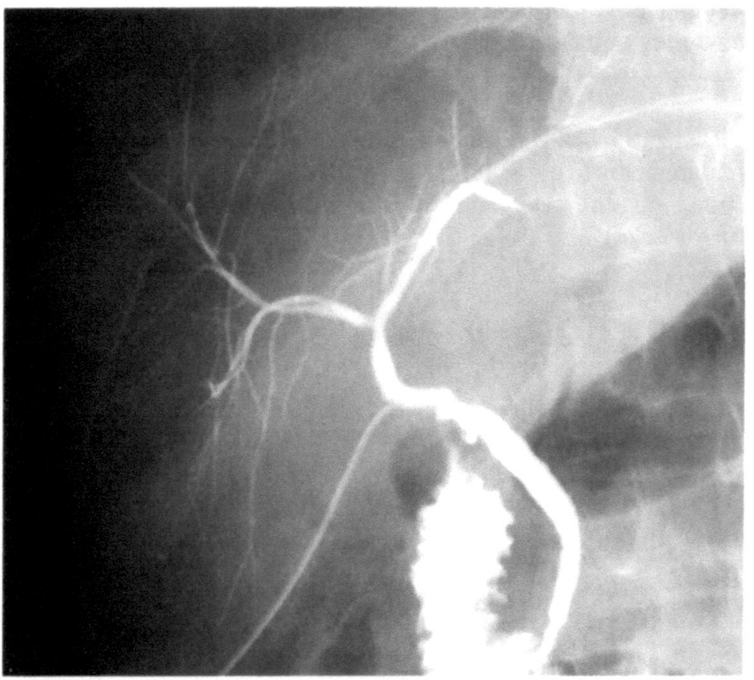

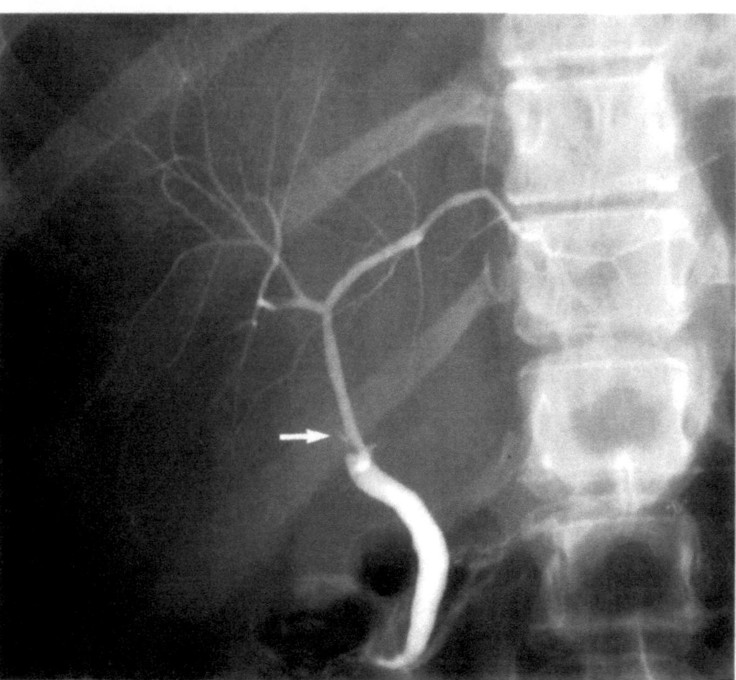

Case 3   Regular Postoperative Anastomosis of the Common Bile Duct of Donor and Recipient

Visualization of the side-to-side choledochocholedochostomy (enlargement) by ERC (Fig. 3). Normal situation with the stump of the recipient's cystic duct after cholecystectomy (*arrowhead*).

Case 4   Normal Cholangiogram After Transplantation of a Reduced-Size Liver Graft

History

A 20-year-old-female patient underwent OLT because of hepatic failure induced by viral infection. When OLT was carried out, the liver transplant had to be reduced in size because of a mismatch between the size of the donor organ and the capacity of the upper right abdominal quadrant. ERC was performed because of cholestasis. Liver histology showed the onset of chronic graft rejection.

ERCP

The cholangiogram reveals a normal caliber of the biliary system of the graft (Fig. 4). Segments V, VI, VII, and VIII have been removed (*clip, arrowheads*). The bile ducts of the donor and recipient are enlarged at the site of end-to-end choledochocholedochostomy. There is no obstruction at the site of the papilla. The pancreatic duct is normal.

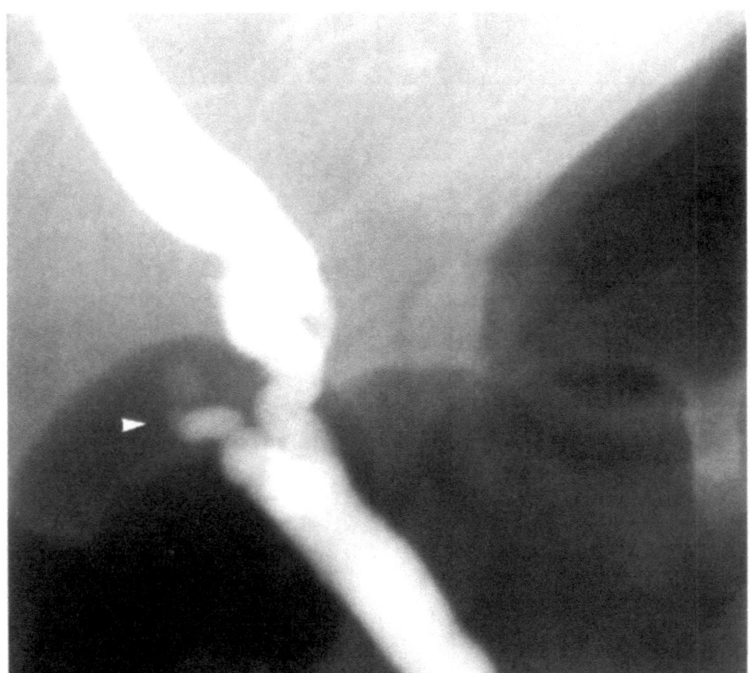

3

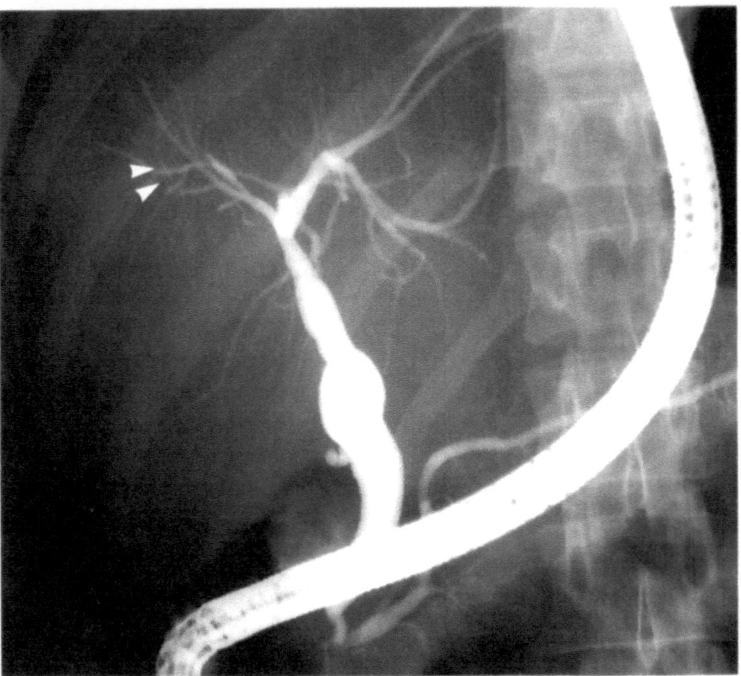

4

Biliary Leakage

Short Overview

Biliary leakage is an early complication following liver transplantation. It is reported to occur in about 5% of cases [1, 7, 30]. About 25% of biliary complications following liver transplantation are caused by leakage. Three different types may be found:

1. Multiple intrahepatic bile extravasations due to diffuse damage to the biliary system [39]. These are usually caused by arterial occlusion or by ischemic-type lesions. The radiologic features are multiple intraparenchymal or perihilar collections of contrast medium. Intrahepatic biliomas may remain clinically inapparent if there is no cholestasis or cholangitis.

2. Following choledochocholedochostomy over a temporary T-tube stent, leakages may occur at the T-tube exit site. Therefore, the total rate of leakages is higher in this type of anastomosis than in that following biliodigestive reconstruction [14, 38, 39]. Leakages at the T-tube exit site are usually not caused by total ischemia of the bile ducts but by local factors such as excessive tension around the T-tube after suture or focal ischemia caused by the suture. Other causes may be irregular placement or partial dislocation of the T-tube. The patients become symptomatic mainly as a result of subhepatic bile collection. If a subhepatic drainage is still in place, additional treatment may not be necessary. Otherwise, surgical or interventional radiological drainage may be required. Closure of the leaking T-tube exit with additional sutures is usually not reliable. The T-tube should always be reopened if still in place. Late T-tube leaks may occur after the removal of the T-tube. If symptoms such as abdominal pain and local or diffuse peritonitis persist for longer than 24 h, nonoperative percutaneous drainage is recommended. With side-to-side bile duct reconstructions which are employed in our department, the anastomosis is splinted by a small calibrated catheter (Cavafix) which is introduced via the cystic duct. In a few cases biliary leaks have occurred at this site and were treated by removal of the catheter. On account of the considerable rate of complications caused by placement of the T-tube, biliary tract anastomosis without the T-tube is recommended [25].

3. Leakage a the site of the bile duct anastomosis [1, 30, 38] is primarily related to surgical technique (75%) or occurs secondary to hepatic artery thrombosis (25%) [7]. Leakage is a serious complication with a mortality rate of up to 48% [13], especially if caused by hepatic artery occlusion. Leaks at this anastomotic site do not appear to be dependent on the chosen type of anastomosis. We have seen comparable rates following side-to-side, end-to-end, and biliodigestive duct reconstruction [29]. Options for surgical repair include drainage, local oversewing, or reanastomosis with conversion of duct-to-duct anastomosis to choledochojejunostomy [31]. Depending on the clinical situation, nonoperative treatment is recommended [10, 33]. The T-tube should be reopened and bile may be diverted by nasobiliary drainage. Percutaneous transhepatic drainage may be required in biliodigestive repair. Internal drainage by means of sphincterotomy and endoscopic stent placement results in an excellent outcome in the treatment of leakage of duct-to-duct anastomoses. In contrast, with hepatic artery thrombosis, many patients are candidates for retransplantation [11, 12, 30, 34, 35].

Case 5 Biliary Leakage After Displacement of a Drainage Catheter and Endoscopic Treatment with Endoprostheses

History

A 59-year-old female patient underwent OLT because of end-stage liver cirrhosis caused by hepatic prophyria. A control check cholangiogram was performed 3 weeks after OLT via a thin drainage catheter (Fig. 5).

Fig. 5a Biliary leakage (*arrow*) is observed at the site of bile duct anastomosis because of the partially displaced drainage catheter. There are air bubbles in the recipient's common bile duct because of catheter displacement. There is no visualization of the biliary tract above the anastomosis. Contrast medium runoff via the papilla is satisfactory.

Fig. 5b ERC reveals a long stenosis at the anastomosis (*arrows*).

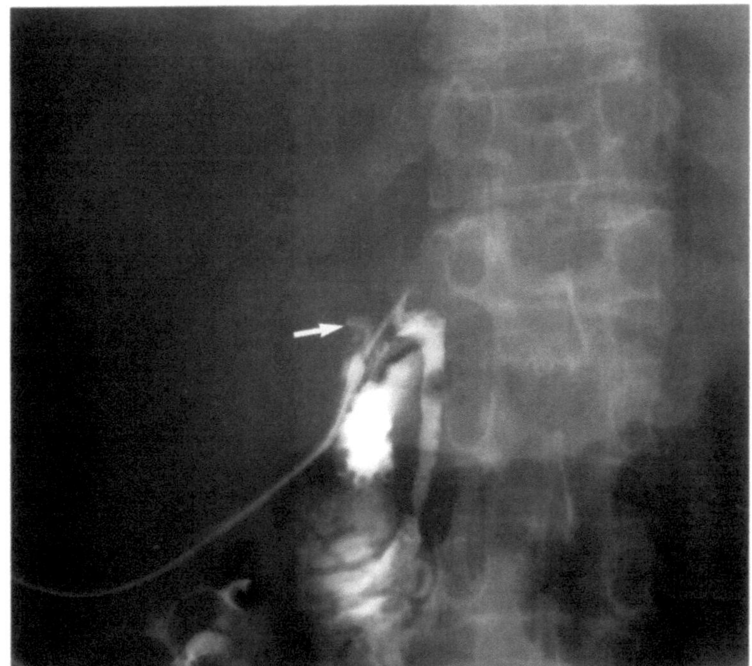

5a

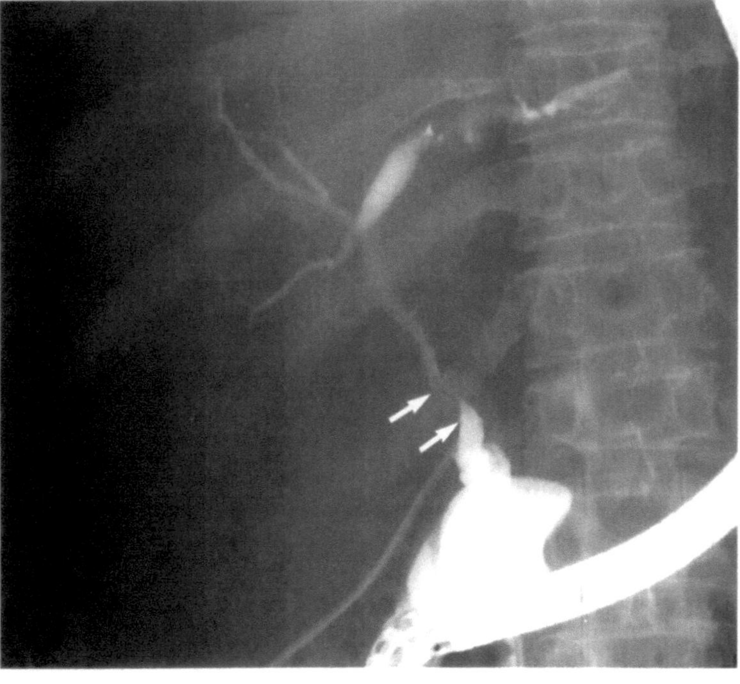

5b

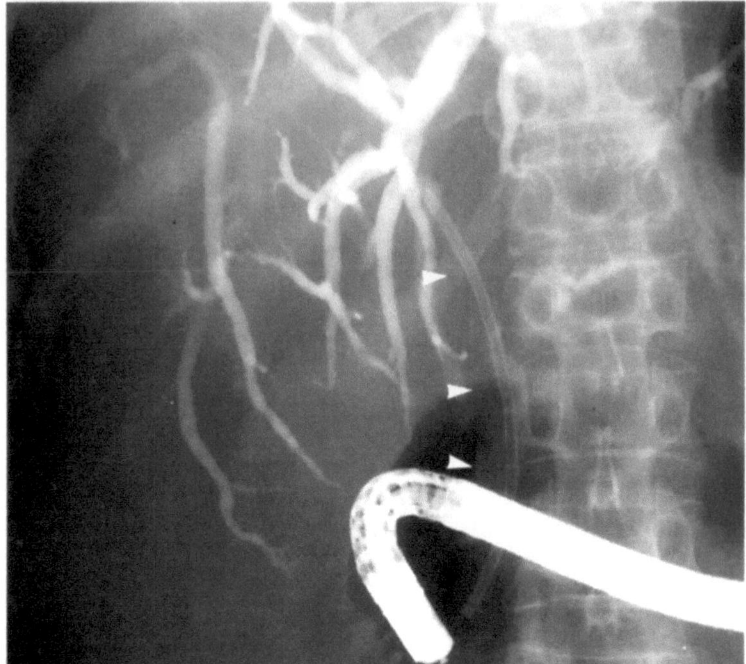

5c

Fig. 5c Endoscopic sphincterotomy and dilation of the stenosis were performed. A 9-cm 8.5F endoprosthesis (*arrowheads*) was placed, resulting in unimpaired bile flow into the duodenum.

Fig. 5d Endoscopic placement of a second endoprosthesis was performed to guarantee a sufficient diameter of the choledochocholedochostomy and to improve bile drainage. Slight aerobilia is seen due to the endoprostheses (*arrowheads*).

Fig. 5e After 6 weeks, both endoprostheses were removed and ERC shows a normal cholangiogram with a normal situation at the site of bile duct anastomosis. No restenosis occurred during 2 years of follow-up.

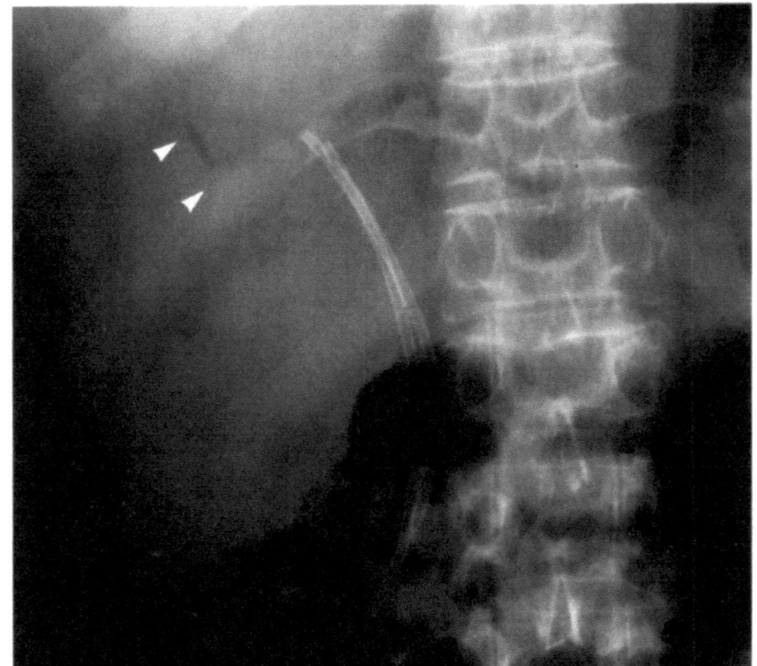

5d

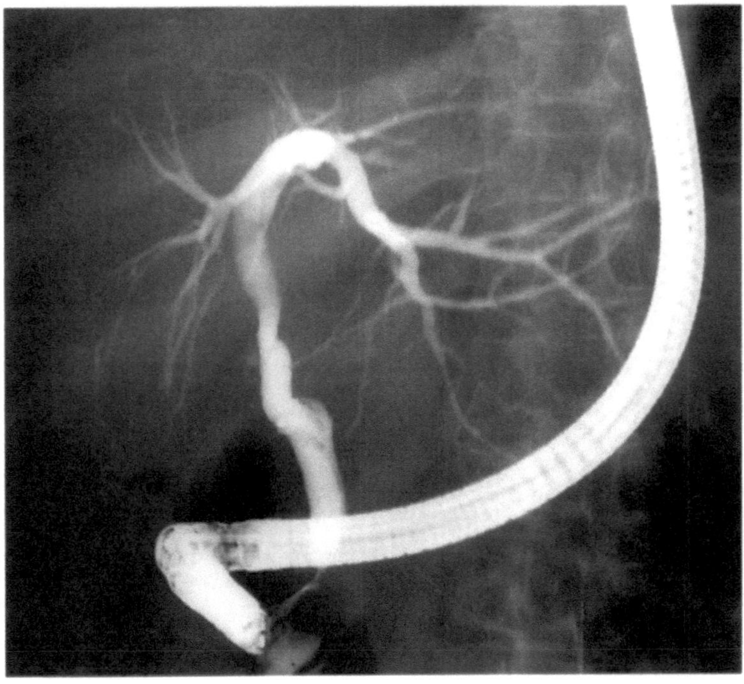

5e

Case 6 Biliary Leakage and Retention of Part of a Disrupted T-Tube; Situation After Endoscopic Removal and Surgical Repair

History

A 27-year-old male patient suffering from galactosemia received a liver graft because of hepatocellular carcinoma. After removal of the T-tube, it was recognized on cholangiogram that one part of the T-shaped drainage had been retained in situ (Fig. 6). The patient therefore developed signs of peritonitis in the right upper quadrant of the abdomen.

Fig. 6a ERC reveals the disrupted part of the T-tube (*arrow*). There is significant bile leakage into the abdominal cavity (*fat arrow*). Endoscopic sphincterotomy was performed and the remaining part of the T-tube successfully extracted. The biliary leak was surgically closed.

Fig. 6b ERC after surgical revision: The stump of the recipient's cystic duct, which was the origin of biliary leakage, was closed by a metal clip (*arrow*). Except for significant kinking of the distal common bile duct, which did not impair bile flow, a normal postoperative cholangiogram is seen.

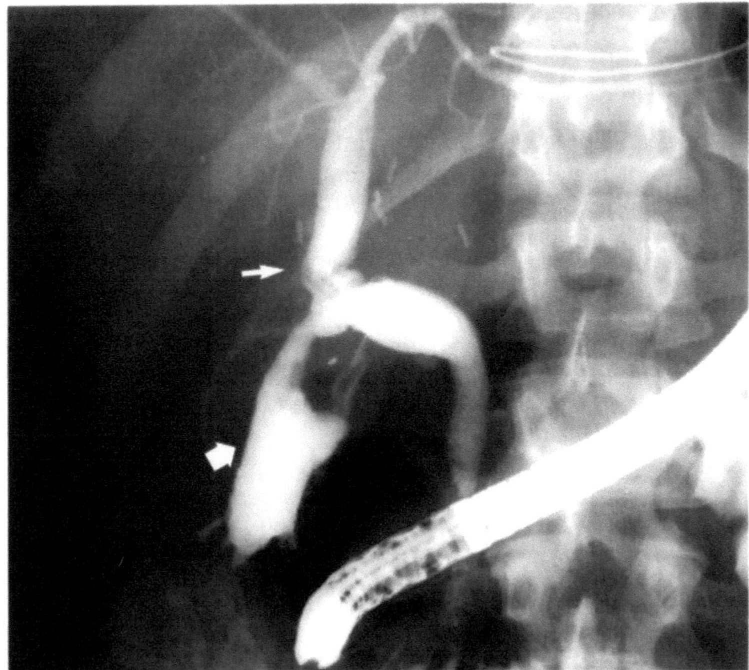

6a

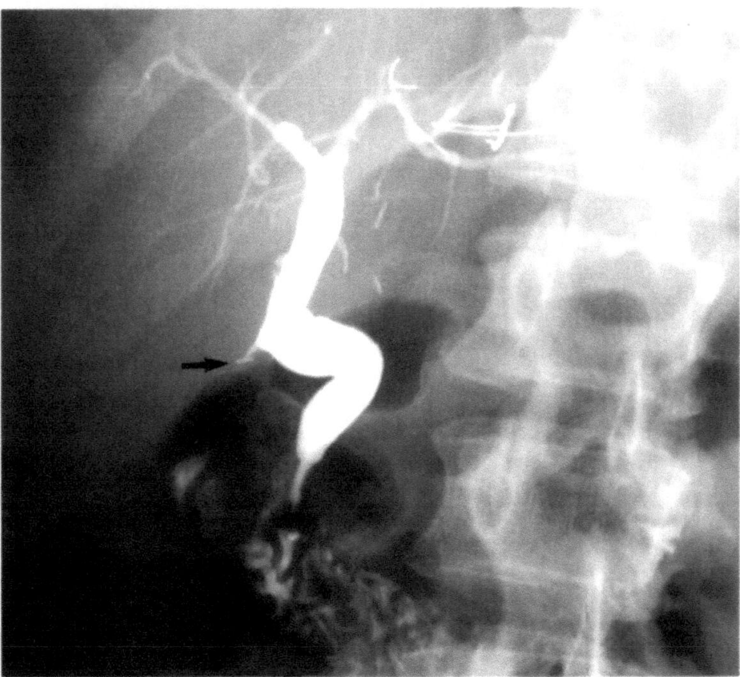

6b

Case 7 Biliary Leakage at the Site of Bile Duct Anastomosis

History
A 63-year-old female patient underwent liver transplantation because of hepatocellular carcinoma. She developed peritonitis 4 weeks after OLT. The ascites fluid contained bile.

ERCP
ERCP shows the graft without a common bile duct (Fig. 7). Both major bile ducts (*arrows*) were anastomosed with the recipient's common bile duct. Slight leakage (*arrowheads*) from the distal part of the recipient's common bile duct was observed. Endoscopic sphincterotomy had to be performed because of sclerosing papillitis. Relaparatomy was necessary as it was not possible to insert an endoprosthesis to seal the site of biliary leakage.

Case 8 Biliary Leakage and Stenosis at the Site of Bile Duct Anastomosis

History
A 49-year-old female underwent OLT because of subacute hepatic failure induced by hepatitis C virus infection. The function of the grafted liver remained normal until she suddenly developed signs of cholestasis and peritonitis $2\frac{1}{2}$ years after OLT.

ERC (Fig. 8)
Stenosis at the site of anastomosis and leakage of contrast material from the proximal end of the recipient's bile duct (*arrows*) are seen. The patient underwent surgical revision and recovered uneventfully.

Comment
Biliary leakage at a late stage after OLT is a very rare and unusual event. No underlying reasons could be discovered.

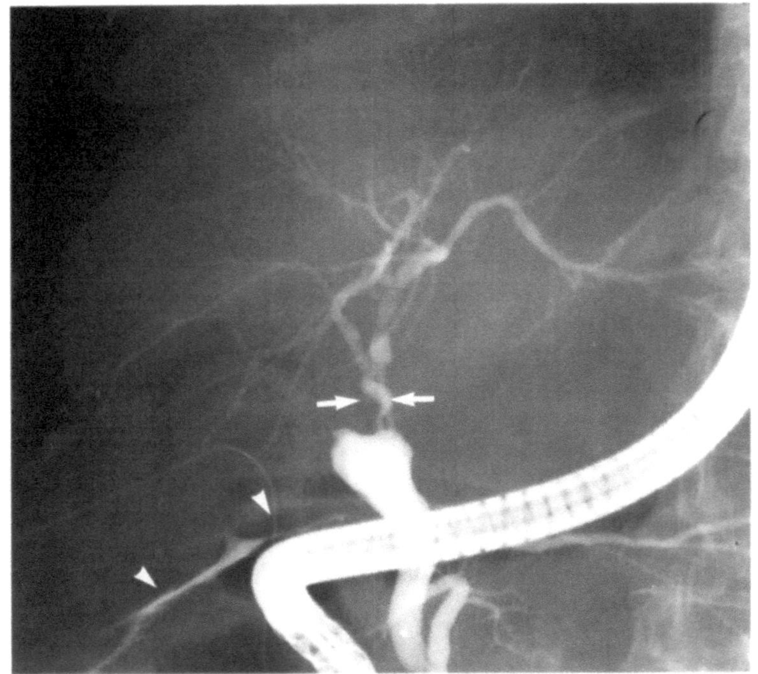

7

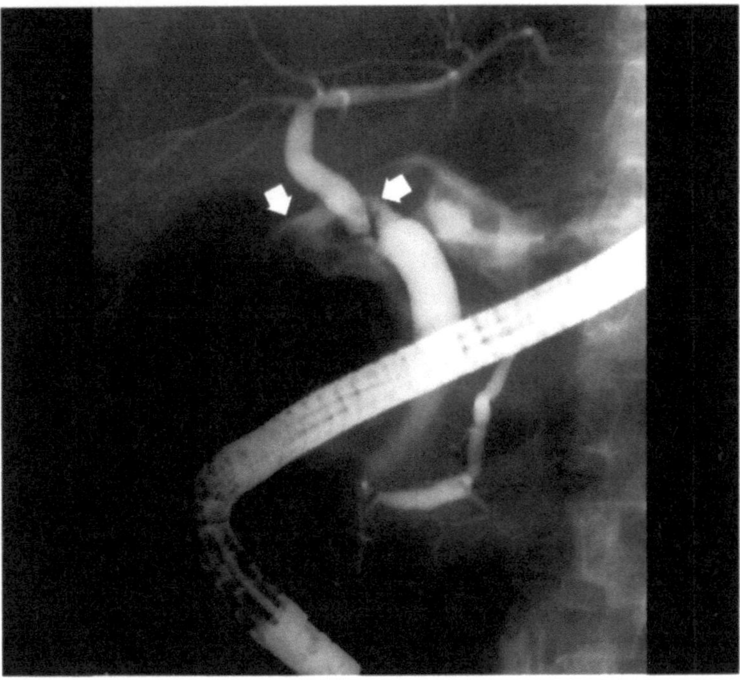

8

Bile Duct Redundancy

Short Overview

Bile duct redundancy is rare and the result of either a donor or a recipient bile duct that is too long. It is normally harmless, leading to an S-shaped common bile duct. Bile flow is usually not impaired, unless severe kinking leads to partial or complete obstruction with subsequent cholangitis [40]. In these cases endoscopic intervention, e.g., placement of metal stents, may be required.

Case 9 Bile Duct Redundancy with Unimpaired Bile Flow

History
A 53-year-old patient who underwent transplantation because of virally induced liver cirrhosis had elevated liver enzymes 10 months after OLT. ERCP and a liver biopsy were performed. The liver histology showed chronic active hepatitis due to serologically proven hepatitis C reinfection.

ERCP (Fig. 9)
Cholangiography revealed a normal intrahepatic biliary system of the liver graft with a slight circular stenosis of the bile duct anastomosis (*arrow*). The recipient's bile duct showed an S-shaped elongation. No further measures were considered necessary after rapid runoff of the contrast medium was observed by fluoroscopy with the patient in supine position and no irregularities of the bile duct system due to cholangitis could be seen.

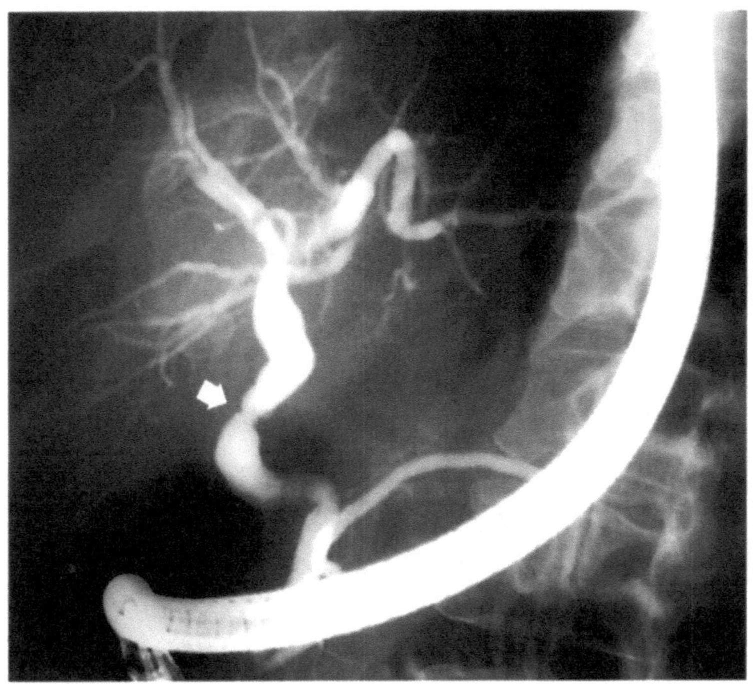

Case 10 Bile Duct Redundancy with Impaired Bile Flow and Subsequent Bacterial Cholangitis; Treatment by Insertion of a Metal Stent

History

A 50-year-old male patient underwent OLT because of end-stage alcohol-induced liver cirrhosis. Examination of the explanted liver revealed a 2-cm hepatocellular carcinoma, which had not been detected previously. Two months after transplantation the patient presented signs of cholestasis.

ERC (Fig. 10)

Fig. 10 a Alteration of the intrahepatic biliary tract is seen with signs of chronic cholangitis. The irregularities in the contrast-filled bile duct system are reminiscent of cellular detritus or pus (*arrowheads*). There were also slight irregularities at the site of anastomosis but no stenosis. Because no changes in the postoperative cholangiograms could be detected, ischemia as the underlying cause is very unlikely. The marked kinking of the bile duct may have impaired the bile flow and led to cholangitis.

Fig. 10 b Endoscopic sphinterotomy was performed and a metal stent (*arrowheads*) was inserted. This procedure straightened out the common bile duct, resulting in improved bile flow. In combination with antibiotic therapy, the cholestasis resolved.

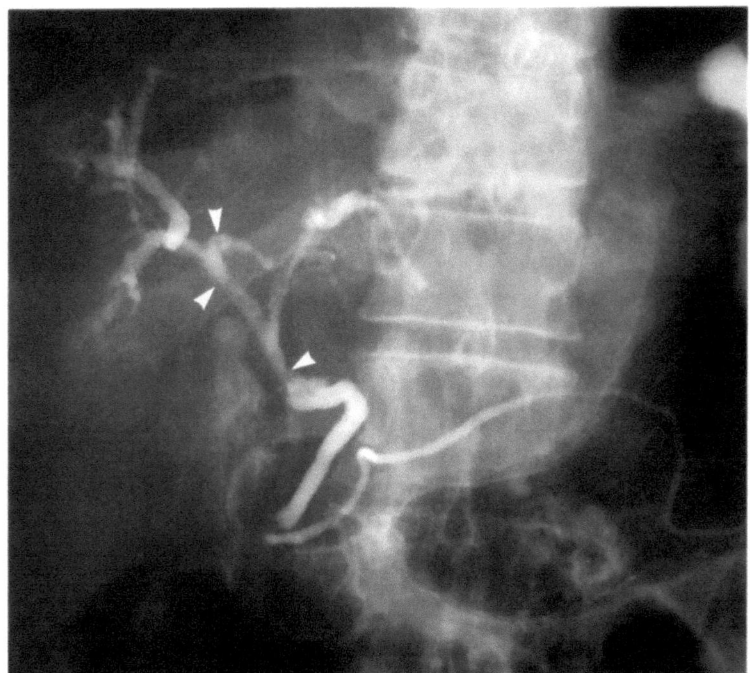

10 a

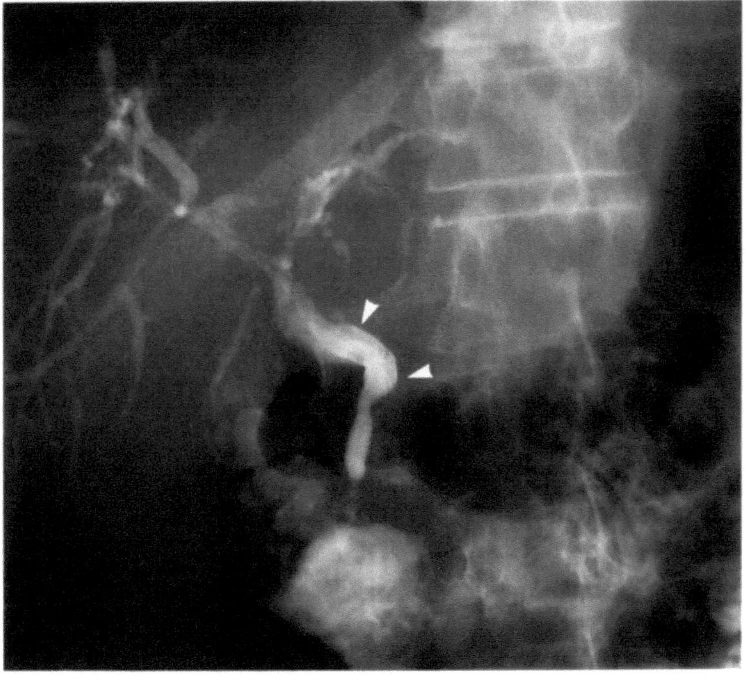

10 b

Sludge in the Biliary System

Short Overview

Sludge formation or even stones in the bile ducts were traditionally thought to be caused by altered bile constituents [18]. However, recent research has shown that biliary strictures are more likely to be the causal factors in sludge and stone formation [10]. Strictures may be followed by biliary stasis and infection which are associated with sludge formation. Additionally, sludge and bile duct casts are often seen in ischemic ducts, especially in grafts with ischemic-type lesions [9, 15, 26]. In ischemic-type lesions, necroses of all layers of the ductal wall may fill the entire lumen of the damaged bile duct. The possible causal factors should always be evaluated before sludge or casts are treated. A solitary stricture may easily be managed by a percutaneous interventional radiological approach; multiple strictures or ischemic-type lesions may, however, be irremediable.

Case 11 Sludge in the Biliary System and Treatment by Balloon Extraction After Sphincterotomy

History
A 49-year-old male patient was transplanted because of end-stage hepatitis B virus-induced liver cirrhosis. ERC was performed 6 months after OLT because of signs of cholestasis (Fig. 11).

Fig. 11a ERC shows nonradiodense floating material (*arrowheads*) in the proximal common bile duct extending into the main left bile duct with an otherwise normal biliary system. Since particles of this material were movable with the catheter within the choledochal duct, sludge was presumed.

Fig. 11b Endoscopic sphincterotomy was performed and the sludge was extracted with a balloon catheter (*arrow*). The film shows that all material had been cleared from the bile ducts.

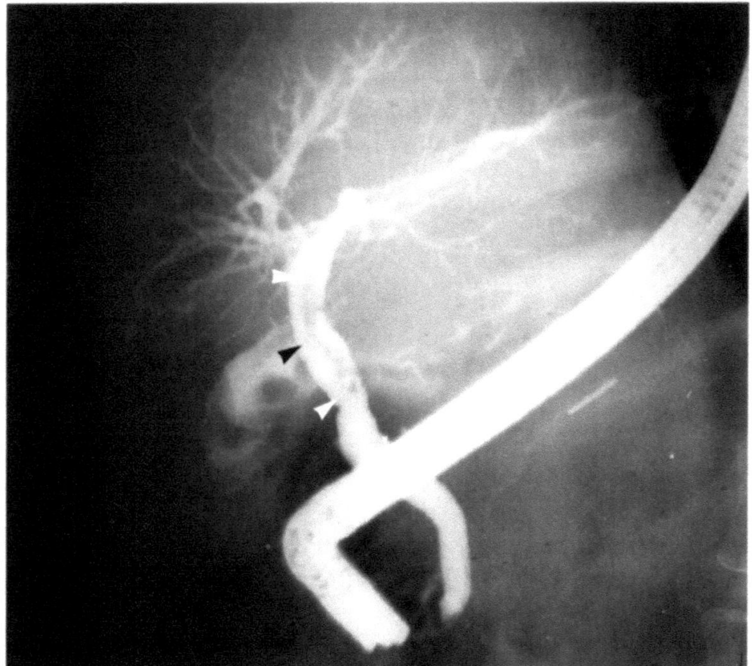

11 a

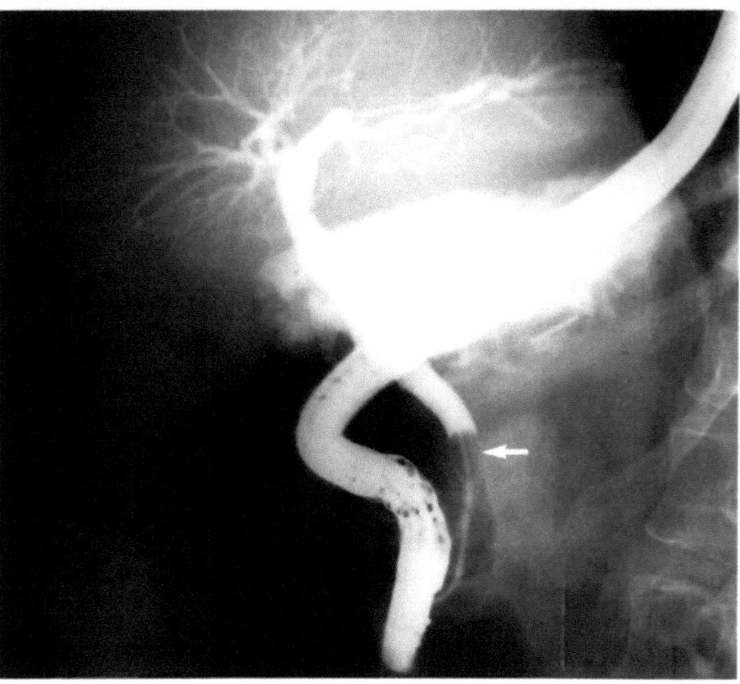

11 b

Stenosis at the Site of Bile Duct Anastomosis

Short Overview

Anastomotic strictures are usually the result of faulty surgical technique or the formation of scar tissue. They occur in 0% [20] to 5% of cases [7, 29]. Whereas in some reports, anastomotic stenoses account for the majority of biliary strictures following liver transplantation [7], our group and other authors found nonanastomotic strictures to be more frequent [23, 26]. Anastomotic strictures occur mainly in the early postoperative period but may also occur later in the course [38]. The type of anastomosis chosen seems to influence this complication. The highest rate of stenosis was found after choledochojejunostomy [2, 7], the lowest, following side-to-side biliary reconstruction [20, 21]. In our experience, side-to-side anastomosis appeared to have the lowest stricture rate but this result was not statistically significant. Finally, arterial thrombosis of the graft has been reported to be a cause of anastomic strictures. In 2 out of 20 patients with anastomotic strictures, hepatic artery occlusion was found [39]. However, this appears to be coincidental and is rather untypical.
In the majority of patients anastomotic strictures of the bile duct require surgical revision [7, 29, 31, 37]. Usually, the choledochocholedochostomy has to be converted to a choledochojejunostomy. A stenotic choledochojejunostomy requires surgical revision. Biliary anastomotic strictures may be treated by balloon dilation. Repeated interventions may be necessary, since the rate of restenosis is high. Long-term patency does not exceed 30%–40% [10]. In our experience endoscopic stenting of the stenotic area by a bile duct prosthesis was beneficial in some patients. Metallic expandable stents should only be used if surgical revision of the anastomosis is not possible.

Case 12   Stenosis at the Site of Bile Duct Anastomosis; Endoscopic Treatment by Dilation and Placement of a Metal Stent

History

A 51-year-old female patient received a liver graft because of chronic hepatic failure due to hepatitis C virus infection. Signs of cholestasis developed 2 months after OLT.

ERC (Fig. 12).

Fig. 12a   ERC demonstrates an approximately 3-cm-long stenotic region at the site of the bile duct anastomosis (*arrowheads*).

Fig. 12b   On the final film the high degree of stenosis is more clearly seen with the patient in supine position.

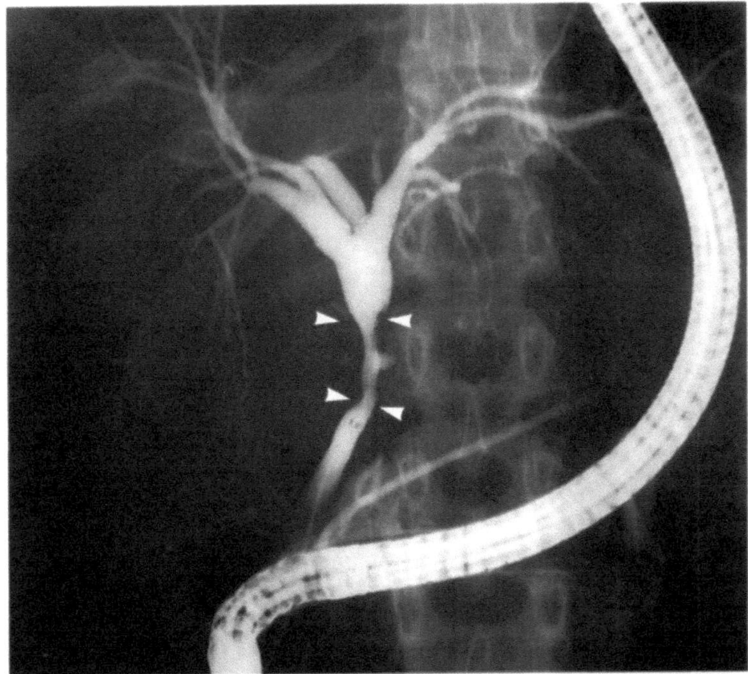

12 a

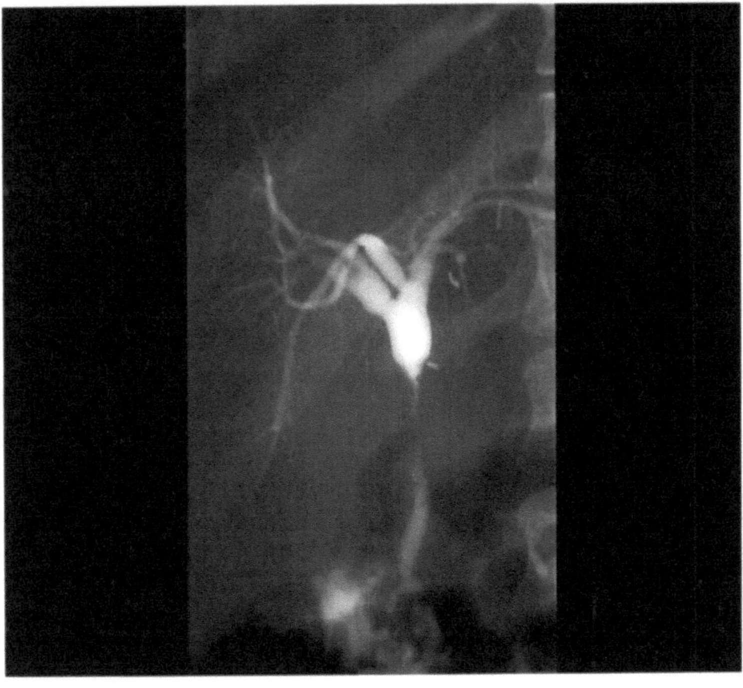

12 b

Fig. 12c   The stenosis was dilated and a balloon-expandable flexible metal stent was inserted. There was good remodelling of the stenosed segment, resulting in good runoff, and the bilirubin level fell to normal values quickly.

Fig. 12d   After 1 year signs of cholestasis redeveloped and the ERC revealed sludge in the stent (*arrowheads*). The stent was dilated and the sludge was removed with a balloon catheter.

Comment

The insertion of permanent stents in benign stenosis is a controversial issue, because these stents cannot normally be removed. Although clogging is unusual because of their large diameter, it can occur, as seen in this patient. In most cases, however, patency of the stent can be restored endoscopically. If this is no longer possible it can be accomplished by percutaneous transhepatic access, which is the alternative but more invasive procedure. In every case, metallic stenting should be performed only if surgical reconstruction is not precluded by this approach.

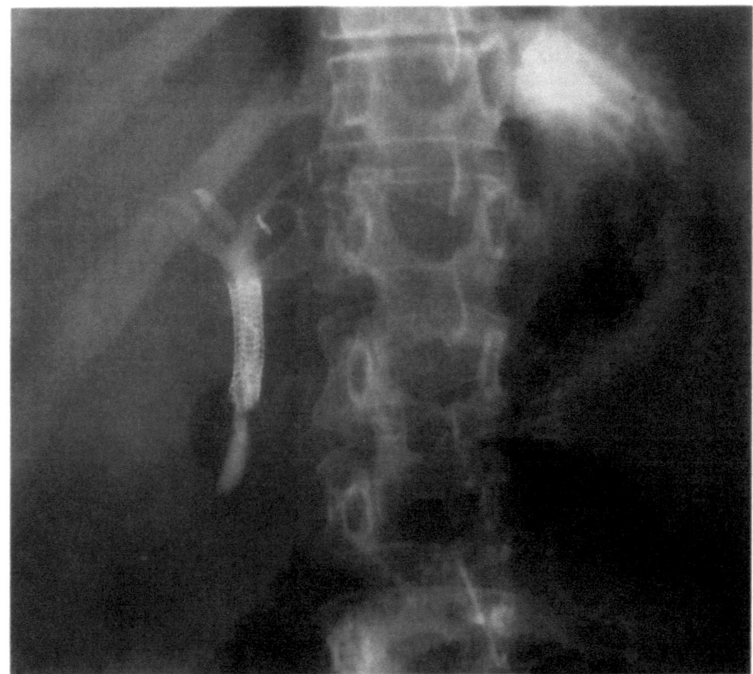

12 c

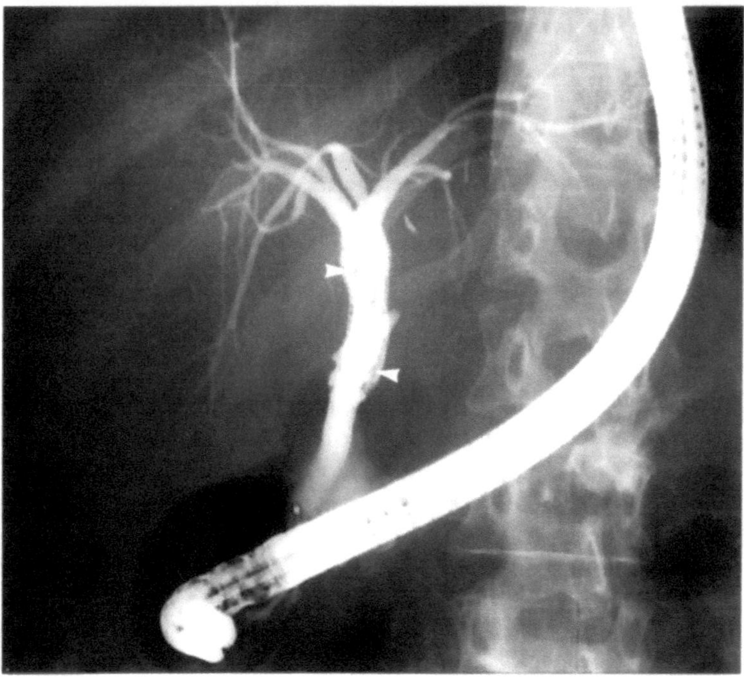

12 d

Case 13 Stenosis at Bile Duct Anastomosis; Treatment by Endoscopic Dilation

History
A 35-year-old male patient underwent liver transplantation because of end-stage liver cirrhosis due to hepatitis B virus infection. A routine postoperative cholangiogram was performed after 2 weeks which showed bile duct stenosis of the site of anastomosis.

Fig. 13 a The biliary system is now visualized by ERC. Stenosis is observed at the site of bile duct anastomosis.

Fig. 13 b Endoscopic sphincterotomy was performed and the stricture was dilated. The figure shows the inflated balloon in position (*arrow*).

Fig. 13 c ERC was performed 3 months later after dilation to visualize possible restenosis at an early stage. No high-grade restenosis could be observed, but there was still a slightly stenotic segment remaining (*arrow*).

Comment
Stenoses which are dilated are reported to have a high rate of recurrence because of elastic recoil of the surrounding tissue. For this reason nonpermanent stents are mainly used to prevent early restenosis due to scarring. Generally, the stents are removed after 3 months. In this case, we refrained from stenting, as dilation was performed early after the operation and we decided to control the diameter of the anastomosis by ERC after 3 months. The clinical and endoscopic follow-up proved to be adequate.

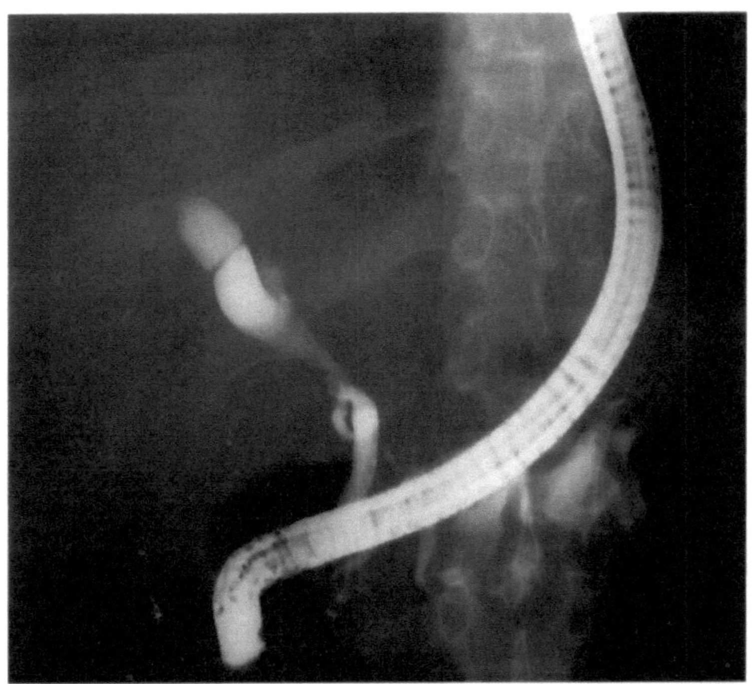

13a

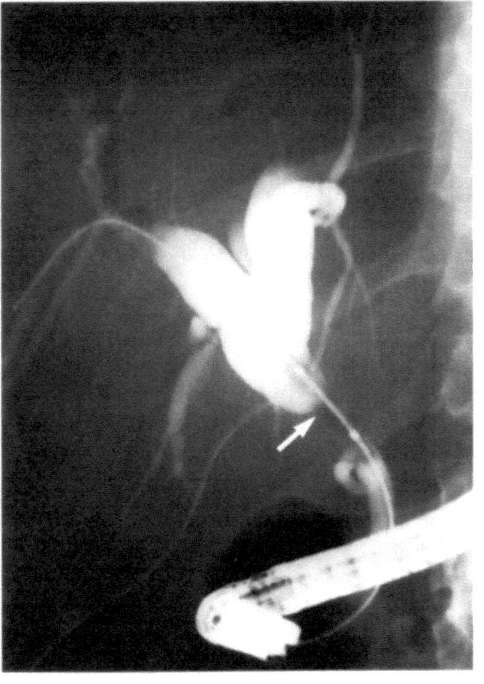

13b

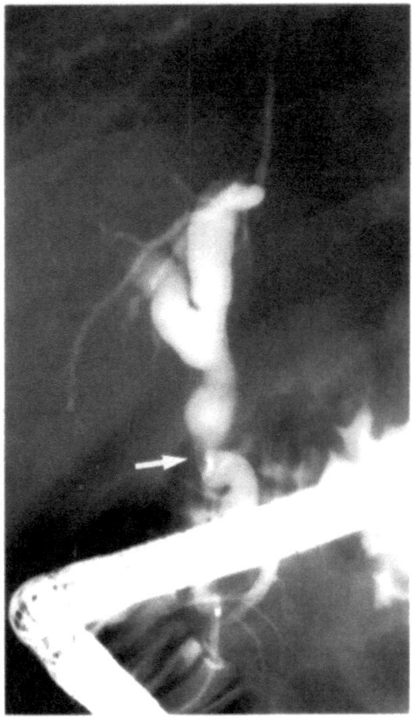

13c

Case 14 Stenosis at the Site of Bile Duct Anastomosis; Endoscopic Treatment by Dilation and Preliminary Insertion of a Plastic Endoprosthesis

History

A 39-year-old female patient underwent transplantation because of hepatocellular carcinoma. Six weeks after OLT, the markers of cholestasis increased and ERC was performed (Fig. 14).

Fig. 14a ERC shows high-grade stenosis at the site of bile duct anastomosis.

Fig. 14b Endoscopic sphincterotomy was performed and the stenosis passed with a guidewire. The stenosis was dilated with a balloon catheter, and the inflated balloon is seen in place (*arrow*).

Fig. 14c After removal of the balloon dilatator the biliary system was visualized and shows a reasonable result. There was still concentric narrowing of the anastomosis (*arrow*).

Fig. 14d To prevent further restenosis, a 8.5 F endoprosthesis was inserted for 3 months.

(Fig. 14c, d see p. 42)

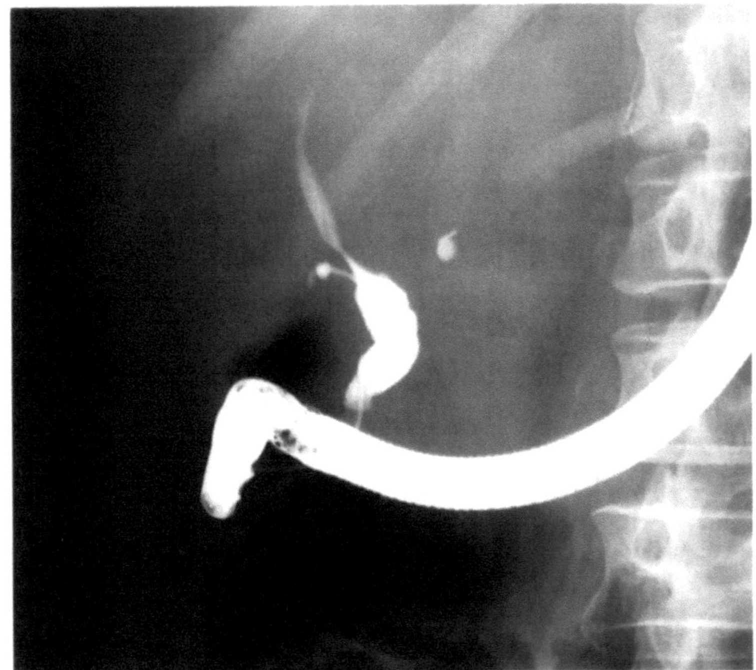

14 a

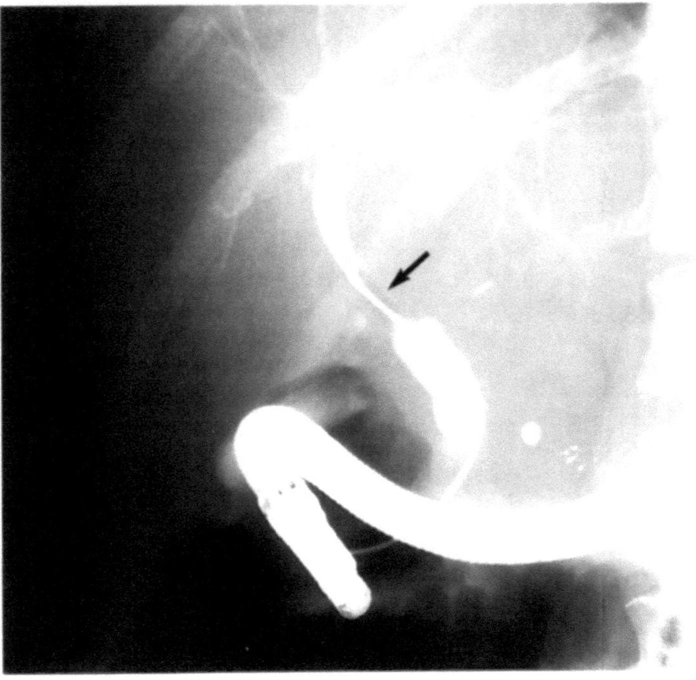

14 b

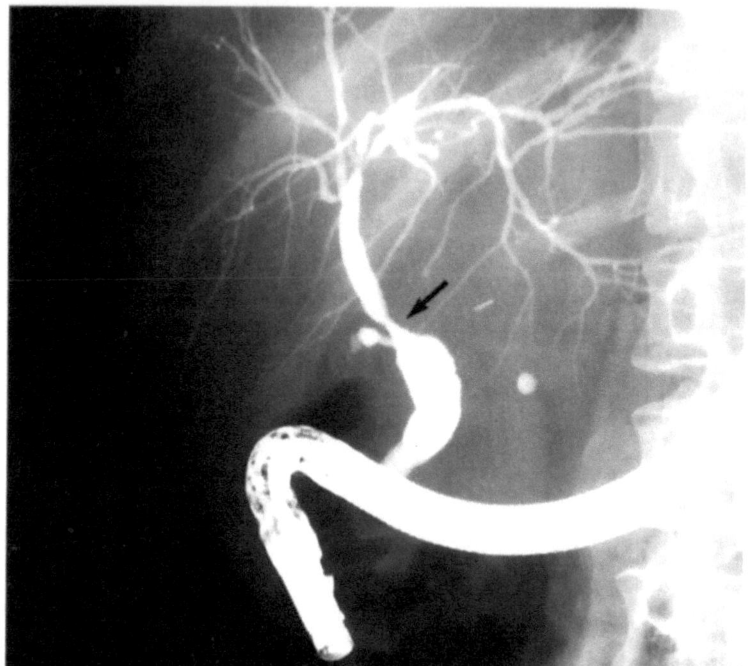

14 c

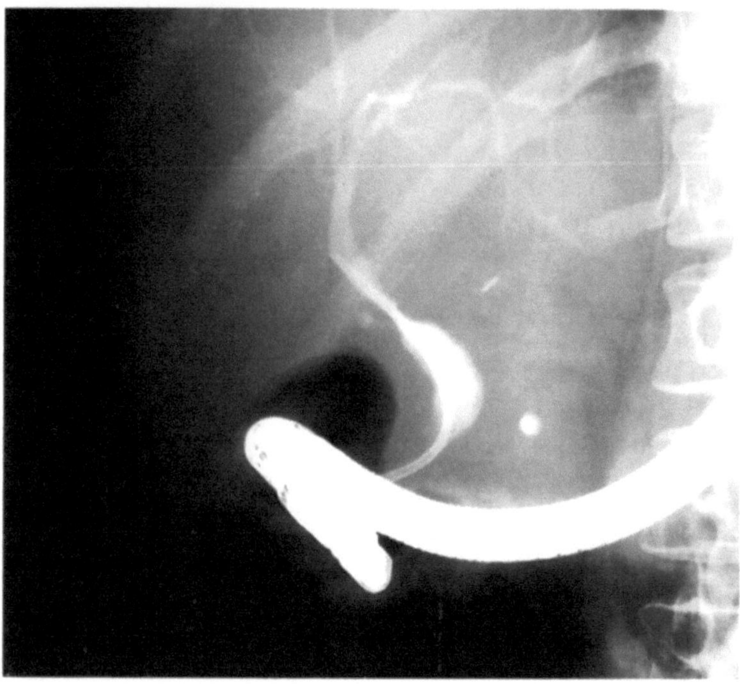

14 d

Bile Duct Stenosis Due to Local Ischemia

Short Overview

Local ischemia may occur in the common bile duct following extensive surgical dissection. The blood supply of the common bile duct is from the right hepatic artery [24, 32]. Damage to small ductal branches results in necrosis and leakage or eventually ductal strictures. Since the anatomy of the blood supply to the bile duct is widely known, this complication should rarely occur nowadays. It requires a hilar reanastomosis. In these case stenting by a prosthesis as a temporary measure may be indicated and advisable.

In left-segment liver transplantation, biliary complications at the site of anastomosis are common sequelae of local ischemia. The blood supply to the central portion of the left bile duct obviously originates from the right hepatic artery. There is no collateral blood supply originating from the left arterial branch [28]. The common bile duct of the segments II and III must therefore be cut step by step until bleeding occurs from the margin, if these segments are to be used for transplantation.

Case 15 Necrosis of the Common Bile Duct and Alteration of the Intrahepatic Ducts

History

A 40-year-old male patient was transplanted because of liver cirrhosis due to hepatitis B virus infection. The postoperative course was uneventful. Four months later an increase of liver enzymes was noted. ERC was performed (Fig. 15). Liver biopsy showed signs of viral hepatitis due to recurrent hepatitis B virus infection.

Fig. 15   ERC shows necrosis of the common bile duct with contrast medium floating around necrotic material (*arrowheads*). There is a minor degree of necrosis of the intrahepatic bile ducts, mainly of the left lobe (segments II and III) with a cavity representing an abscess (*arrow*).

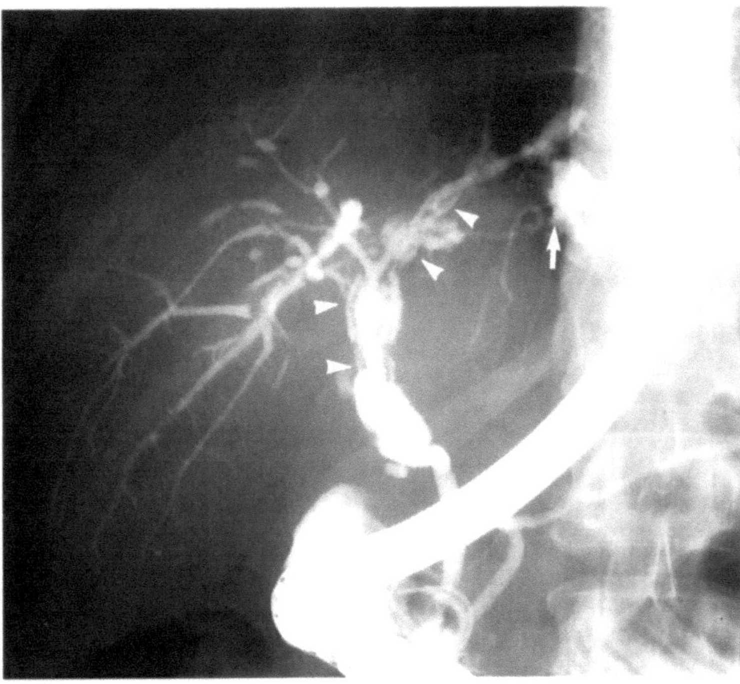

15

Comment

Bile duct alterations are probable due to cold ischemia lasting longer than 13 h. This patient was treated with antibiotics. In the fourth year after transplantation he presented with elevated transaminases and chronic active viral hepatitis. Alkaline phosphatase and gamma-glutamyltransferase were only twice the upper limit of normal and bilirubin was within the normal range. This proves that, despite alterations in the biliary system, the excretory function of the graft may not be severely compromised.

Case 16 Sequelae of Ischemia of the Common Bile Duct of the Grafted Liver

History

A 50-year-old patient received a liver transplant because of cryptogenic liver cirrhosis followed by severe encephalopathy. After 14 months he showed a slight increase in cholestasis markers.

ERC (Fig. 16)

Fig. 16a The ERC shows the sequelae of ischemia of the common bile duct and the distal portion of the right hepatic duct of the graft. Contrast medium is seen flowing around the sludge (*arrowheads*).

Fig. 16b This is shown more clearly in the enlargement. The patient received antibiotic and ursodeoxycholic acid therapy, and cholestasis markers returned to normal levels within 1 month and remained normal for the following 3 years. A further ERC done 1 year later revealed an identical situation.

Comment

Again, this patient demonstrates that despite severe alterations of the main bile duct and bifurcation, a stable condition with regular bile flow via the affected ducts can be observed.

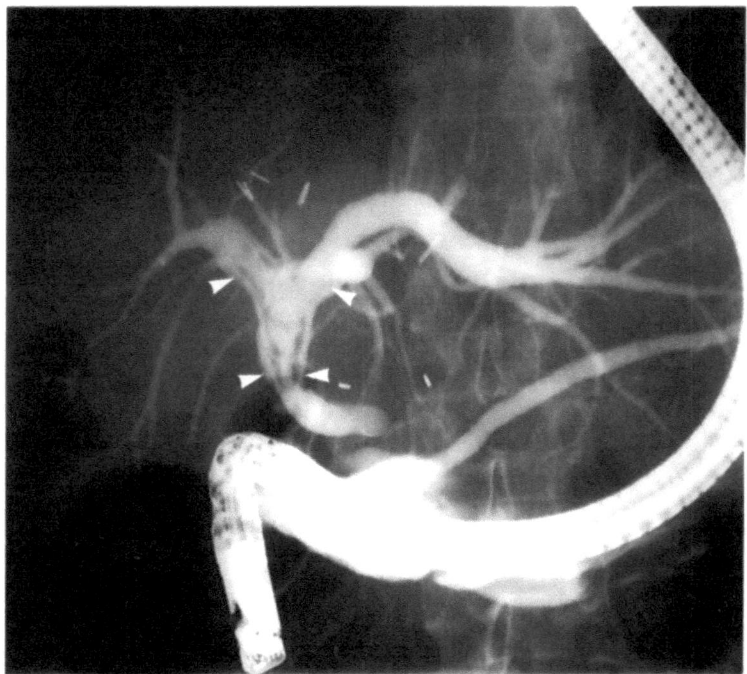

16 a

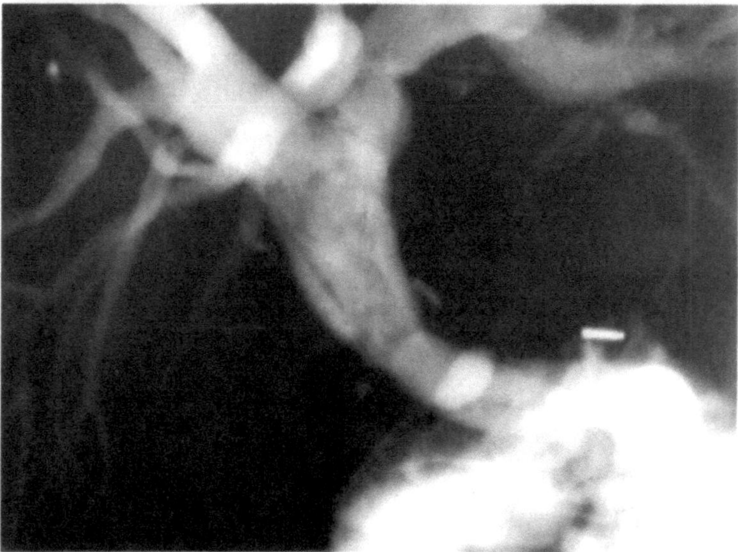

16 b

Case 17 Stenoses of the Main Hepatic Bile Ducts; Endoscopic Treatment

History

A 65-year-old patient underwent liver transplantation because of hepatitis C virus-induced liver cirrhosis.

Cholangiography (Fig. 17)

Fig. 17a A routine cholangiogram performed 3 weeks after OLT via the T-tube is shown. There are marked necroses of the common bile duct and the major intrahepatic ducts (*arrow*) combined with sludge. No further interventional measures were performed at this point. The patient recovered uneventfully from OLT but reinfection with hepatitis C virus occurred. Six months after OLT, liver biopsy showed chronic persistent hepatitis. Transaminases fell to the normal range, but 10 months after OLT, they rose again. Liver histology still showed signs of chronic persistent hepatitis. An ERC was performed.

Fig. 17b ERC was done 10 months after OLT with an inflated balloon catheter to inject contrast material at a certain pressure. Stenoses (*arrowheads*) of all major bile ducts as well as the common bile above the anastomosis were seen. Moreover, there were signs of necrosis and minor sludge particles.

(Fig. 17c–f see p. 50, 51)

Comment

The stenoses of the major bile ducts in this patient were obviously due to local ischemia. All bile ducts were successfully dilated. On follow-up, the patient experienced restenosis every 8 to 9 months. Until now he has had to undergo redilatation four times. In two cases these procedures were performed in one session and in two instances on an outpatient basis. It is of interest that the patient never showed elevation of cholestasis markers, but rather elevation of transaminases, when restenosis had occurred.

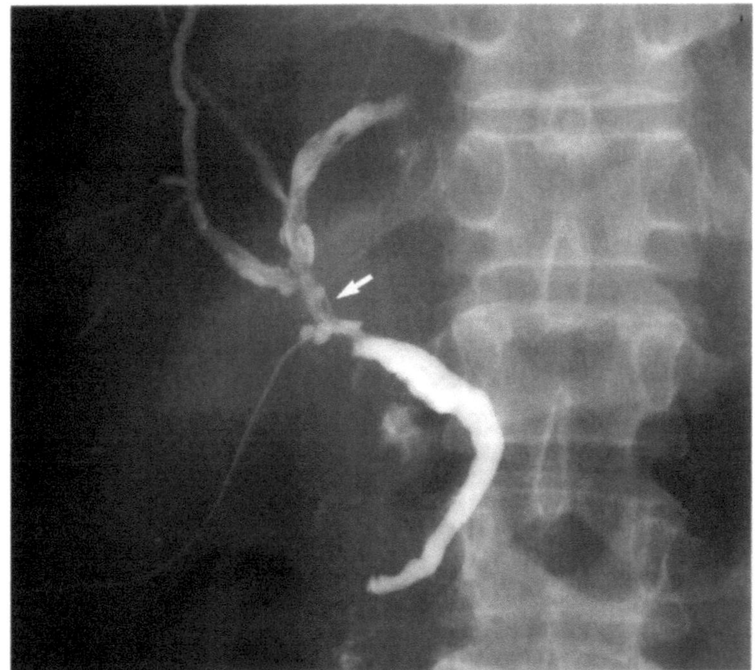

17 a

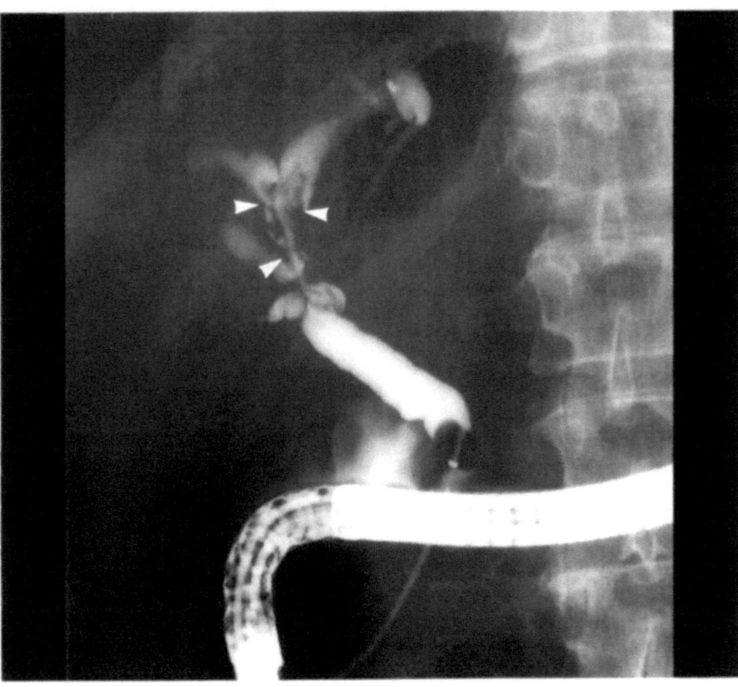

17 b

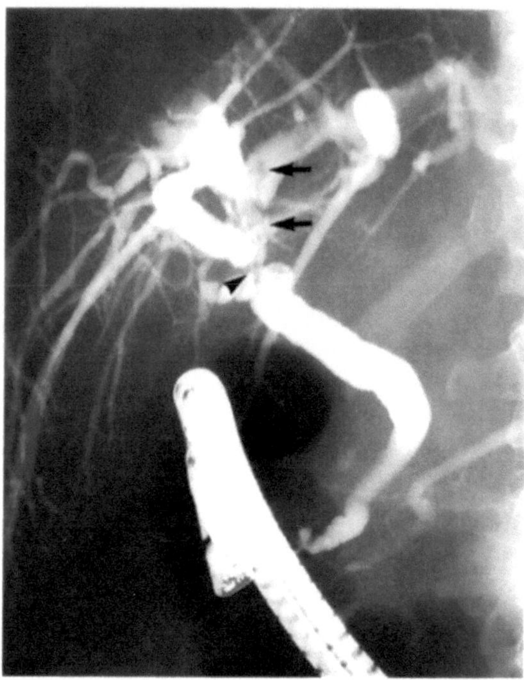

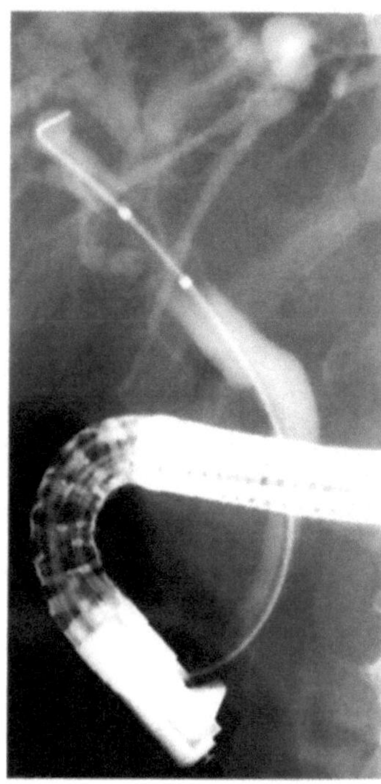

17 c   17 d

Fig. 17 c The intrahepatic ducts are filled and the extrahepatic bile ducts distal to the concentric short stenotic common bile duct of the donor (*arrowhead*) have normal calibers and no signs of inflammation, but sludge is present in the bile ducts at the bifurcation and mainly in the left hepatic duct (*arrows*).

Fig. 17 d All three bile ducts were intubated sequentially with a guide wire and dilated with a balloon. Dilation of the right hepatic duct is shown with the inflated balloon in place.

Fig. 17 e The guide wire is placed through an uninflated balloon catheter into the left hepatic main duct prior to dilation.

Fig. 17 f The final check cholangiogram after dilation demonstrated a fairly good result. There is still some sludge in the bifurcation and the upper part of the common bile duct (*arrow*).

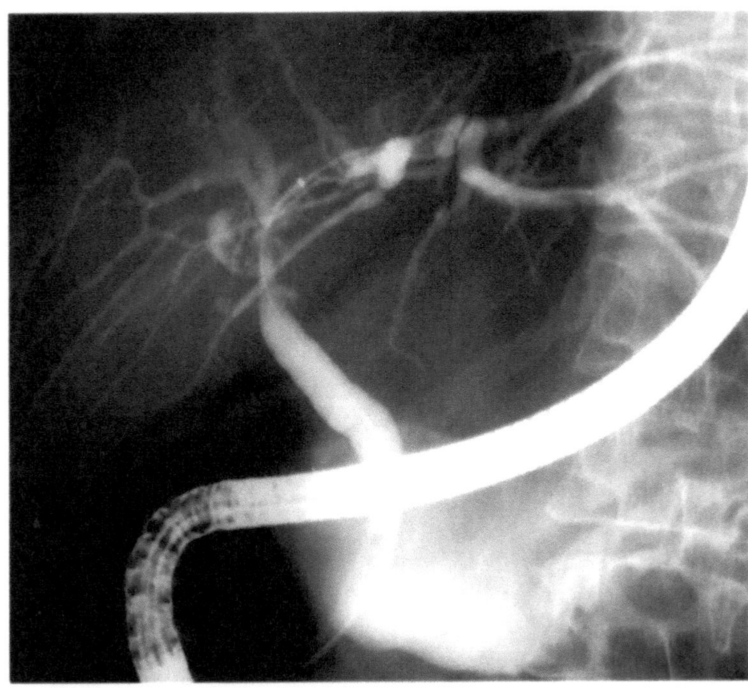

17 e

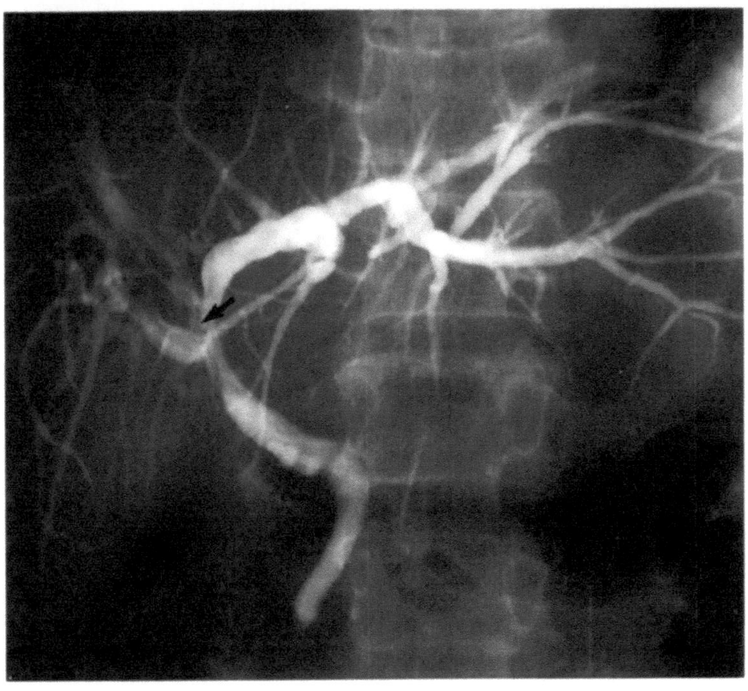

17 f

Case 18 Stenoses of All Major Bile Ducts Following Ischemia

History
A 56-year-old patient had received a liver transplant because
of hepatocellular carcinoma. The postoperative course was uneventful. Eleven months later he presented with signs of cholestasis.

ERC (Fig. 18)
ERC shows the sequelae of local ischemia. Stenoses of all major ducts (*arrowheads*) in the liver hilum and necrosis of the
common bile duct are observed. Three of the stenoses were
passed with a rigid 5 F dilatator after a guide wire had been
advanced in each bile duct. After dilation, the signs of cholestasis disappeared and are still absent after 3 years of follow-
up.

Comment
The cause of the stenoses is probably local ischemia. It is note-
worthy that it was confined to the liver hilum. As the extrahepatic common bile duct was only slightly involved and arterial
occlusion had been excluded by angiography, the origin of this
local impairment of blood supply remains uncertain.

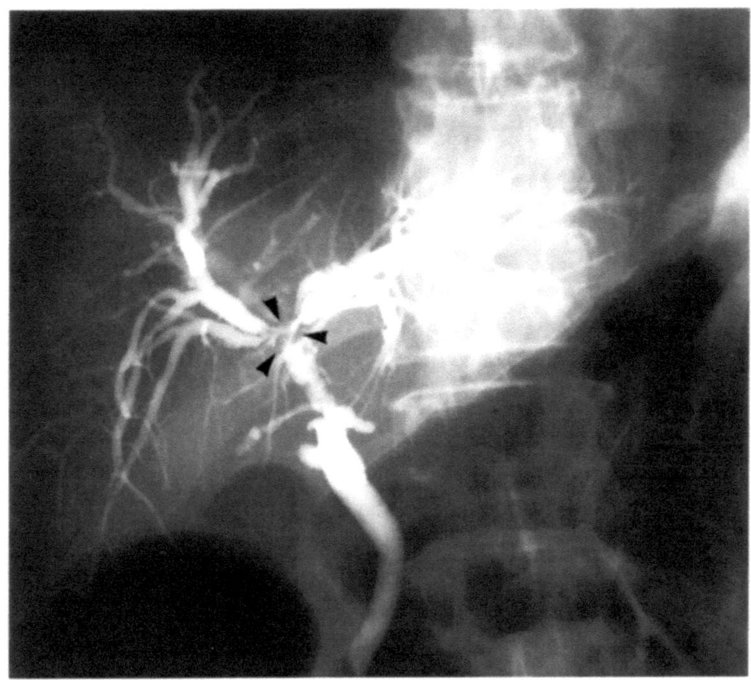

18

Ischemic-Type Lesions Following Long Cold Ischemia

Short Overview

Ischemic-type lesions are a special type of bile duct lesion without obvious underlying causes such as hepatic artery thrombosis, blood group nonidentity, chronic rejection, or severe ascending cholangitis due to anastomotic strictures. Ischemic-type lesions are characterized by multiple strictures and dilatations involving the biliary tree of the graft. Nonanastomotic strictures without obvious causes have been described previously by several authors [8, 37, 39]. This complication, however, was not identified as a particular entity prior to 1992 [9, 15, 26]. Ischemic-type lesions have been found in up to 19% of cases [26], and they are significantly associated with a preservation time exceeding 10 to 12h. Remarkably, this complication was rarely seen during the era when preservation was performed with Collins' solution [15].
The high viscosity of the University of Wisconsin solution may contribute to the development of this complication.

Ischemic-type lesions have been differentiated in two types [33]:

Type A: Total (extrahepatic and intrahepatic) involvement of the biliary tree of the graft
Type B: Involvement of the extrahepatic biliary ducts including the bile duct bifurcation.

Type A lesions occurred in the majority of patients (ratio type A:type B = 2.5:1) [33]. Retransplantation is indicated in many patients with type-A lesions. Endoscopic and percutaneous treatment may be palliative approaches. These include balloon dilation, stenting, or rinsing. In type-B lesions percutaneous interventional procedures may be the treatment of choice [23, 27, 33].

Case 19 Alterations of the Intra- and Extrahepatic Biliary System After OLT; Follow-Up Studies

History
A 65-year-old patient underwent liver transplantation because of liver cirrhosis. Six weeks after OLT, alkaline phosphatase and gamma-glutamyl-transferase were increased and a cholangiogram was performed (Fig. 19).

Fig. 19 a Cholangiogram via the thin drainage catheter: Profound alterations of both intra- and extrahepatic bile ducts are seen. There was necrosis of the common bile duct of the graft as well as narrowing and dilation (*fat arrows*) of the intrahepatic ducts. In addition, there is filling of suspected small abscesses, mainly in the right liver lobe (*arrows*).

Fig. 19 b ERC which allows better filling of the intrahepatic biliary system was performed after a further 6 weeks, revealing no marked improvement. There is stenosis of the right and left intrahepatic ducts with marked dilation of peripheral segment branches.

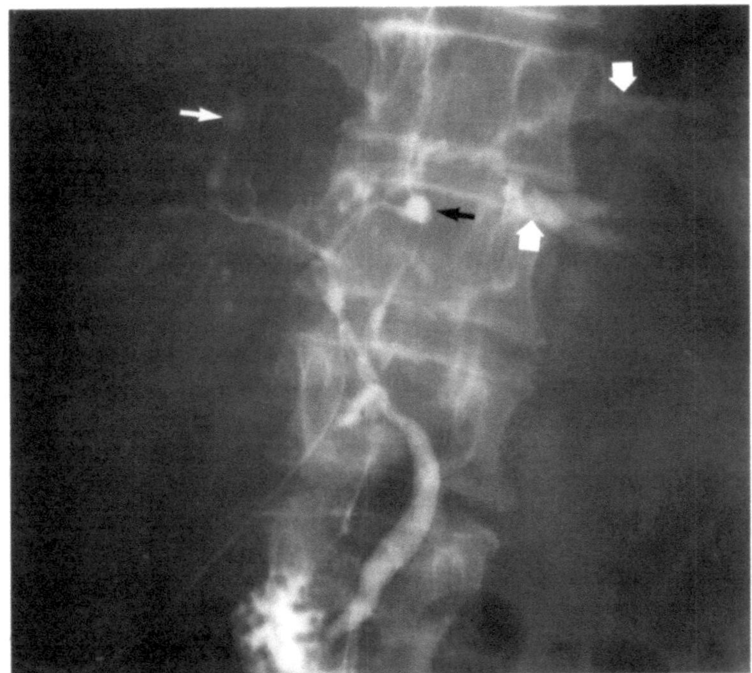

19 a

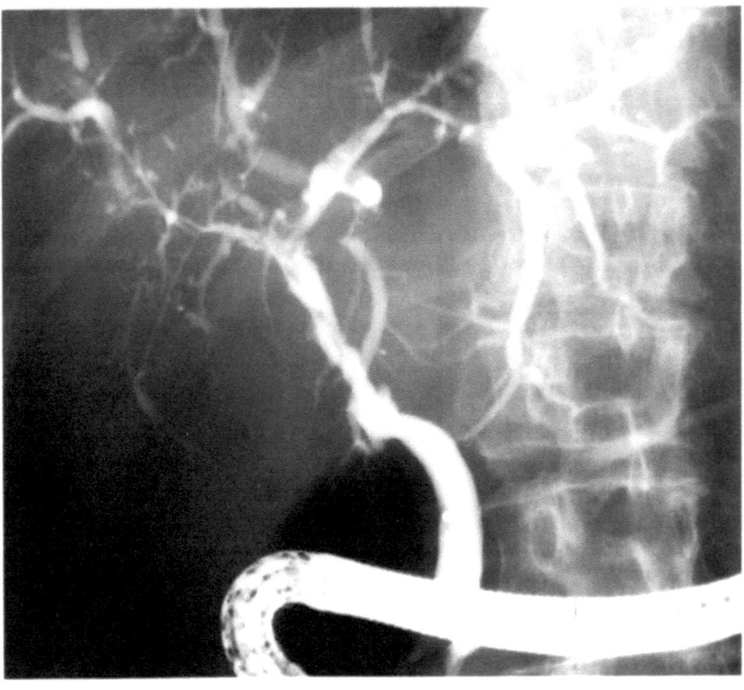

19 b

Fig. 19c Cholangiogram taken 1 min after filling of the system. The patient is in the suspine position and the contrast medium runs off quickly despite the alterations of the biliary tract.

Comment

Alterations of the biliary tract in this patient are probably due to prolonged cold ischemia of the graft after harvesting, which in this case was longer than 12h. Other causes, e.g., occlusion of the hepatic artery, were excluded by angiography.

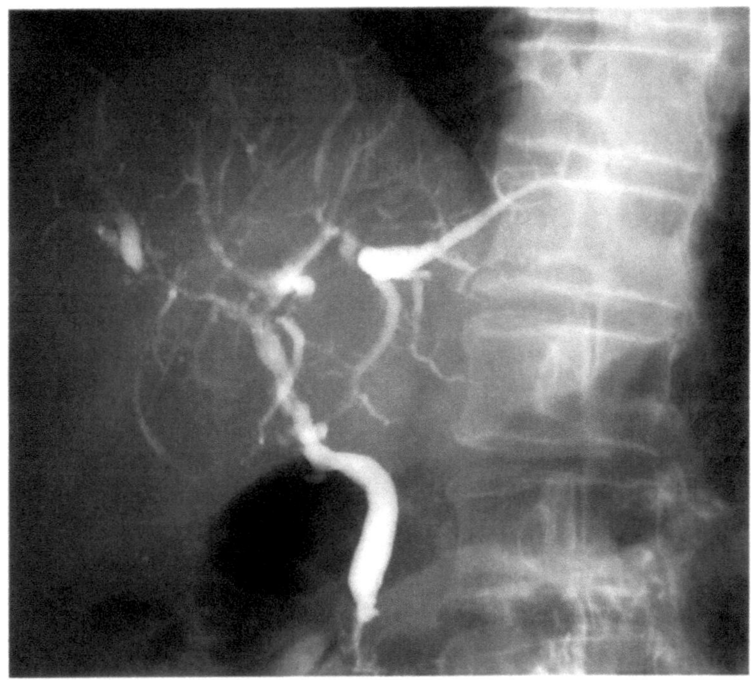

19 c

Case 20 Severe Alterations of the Intra- and Extrahepatic Biliary System; Endoscopic Treatment and Follow-Up Films

History
A 25-year-old female patient received a liver graft because of acute liver failure of unknown origin. After 8 months, she developed signs of cholestasis.

Cholangiography (Fig. 20)

Fig. 20a Necroses proximal to the site of the choledochocholedochostomy of the intrahepatic biliary tract are seen combined with multiple stenoses of the intrahepatic bile ducts (*arrowheads*).

Fig. 20b The common hepatic bile duct and the main left bile duct were dilated. The figure shows the deflated balloon in position. Cholestasis markers fell with an alkaline phosphatase remaining at 1.5 times the upper limit and gamma-glutamyltransferase at 3 times the upper limit of normal.

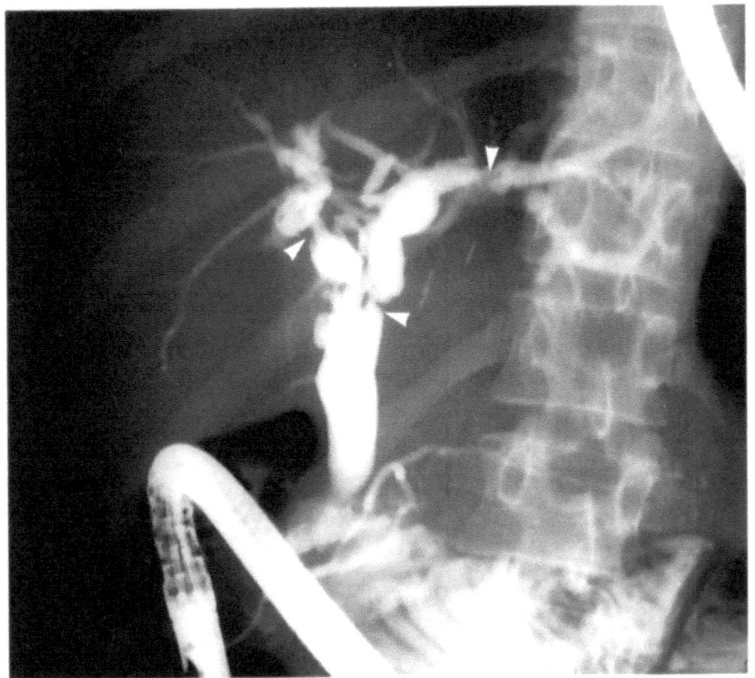

20 a

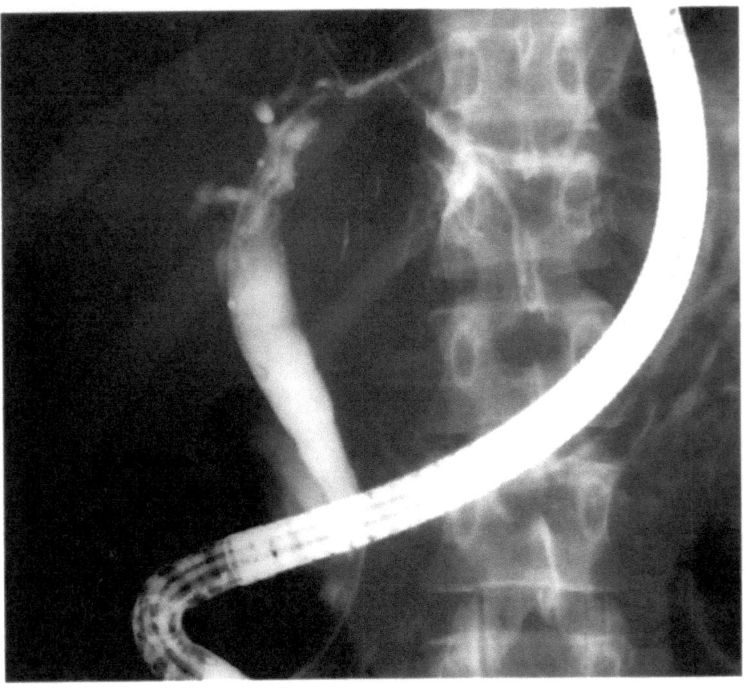

20 b

Fig. 20 c On a check ERC taken 4 years later, stenoses of the extrahepatic bile duct (*arrow*) and of the left liver lobe are visible. The patient developed high-grade concentric anastomotic stenosis. There is atrophy of the right liver lobe and an enlargement of the left liver lobe (segments II and III) because the biliary duct extends far into the left upper quadrant of the abdomen, which signifies a compensatory hypertrophy of the left lobe (*fat arrows*). There is no visualization of the biliary tract of the right liver lobe.

Comment

Cold ischemia time in this patient amounted to 13 h. After 4 years the right hepatic biliary system can no longer be visualized. Surprisingly, no cholestasis of the right hepatic system was seen on ultrasound. The patient refused to undergo endoscopic procedures to restore bile flow from the hepatic system, and markers for cholestasis were only slightly elevated (see above).

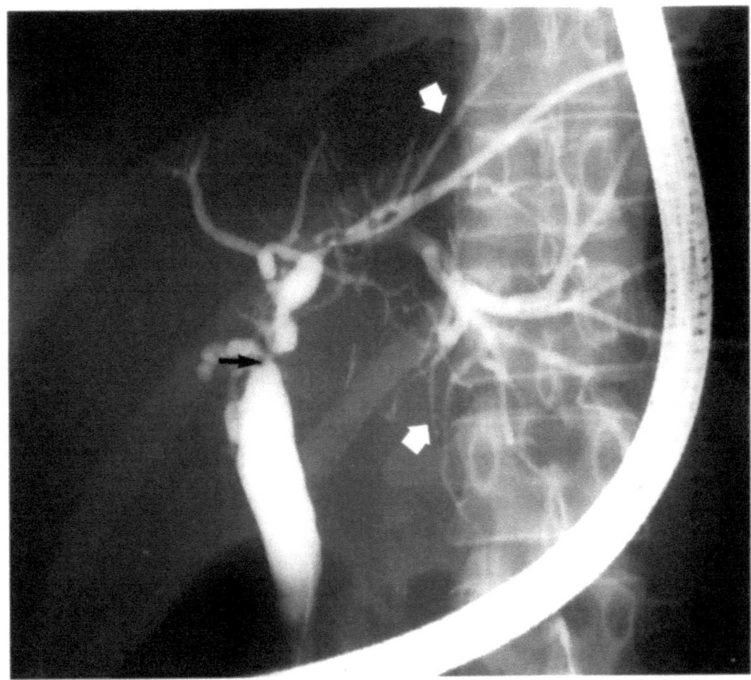

20 c

Case 21 Progressive Sequelae from Prolonged Cold Ischemia

History
A 32-year-old male patient underwent liver transplantation because of alcohol-induced liver cirrhosis. Markers of cholestasis increased after 2 months.

ERC (Fig. 21)

Fig. 21a ERC performed 2 months after OLT showed alterations of the intrahepatic biliary system with narrowing and multiple stenoses *(arrows).*

Fig. 21b ERC taken 15 months after OLT shows marked progression of the alterations of the intrahepatic ducts and obliteration of smaller ducts.

Comment
Because of the clinical course, the alterations are probably due to a prolonged cold ischemia time rather than to chronic graft rejection. As the bilirubin was in the normal range and the alkaline phosphatase and gamma-glutamyltransferase levels were stable at three times the upper limit of normal, the patient was followed on an outpatient basis. At present, he does not require retransplantation because of his stable clinical condition.

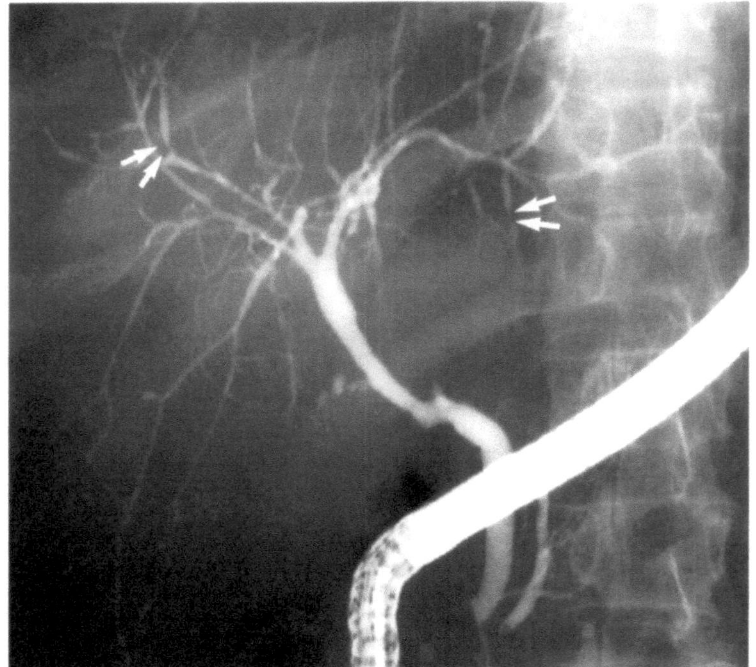

21 a

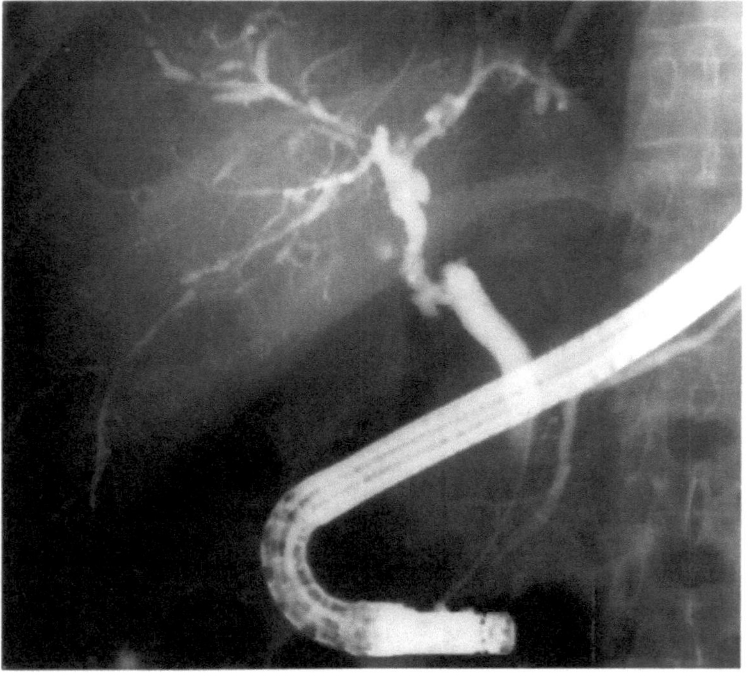

21 b

Case 22   Course of Ischemic-Type Biliary Lesions

History
A 42-year-old patient had received a liver transplant because of alcohol-induced liver cirrhosis.

Cholangiography (Fig. 22)

Fig. 22a   Routine cholangiogram 8 weeks after OLT shows signs of an ischemic-type biliary lesion with short concentric stenoses in the main right and left bile duct (*arrowheads*). Cold ischemia time was 14h.

Fig. 22b   The left main hepatic duct is visualized by ERC 4 months after OLT. There are circumscript concentric stenoses, irregular outlines of the bile ducts, and some marginal spaces in the visualized biliary tree as signs of necroses and sludge (*fat arrows*). There is only incomplete visualization of the right main bile duct system.

Comment
The patient had normal bilirubin levels and only a slight elevation of the other cholestasis markers. He has been followed up on an outpatient basis.

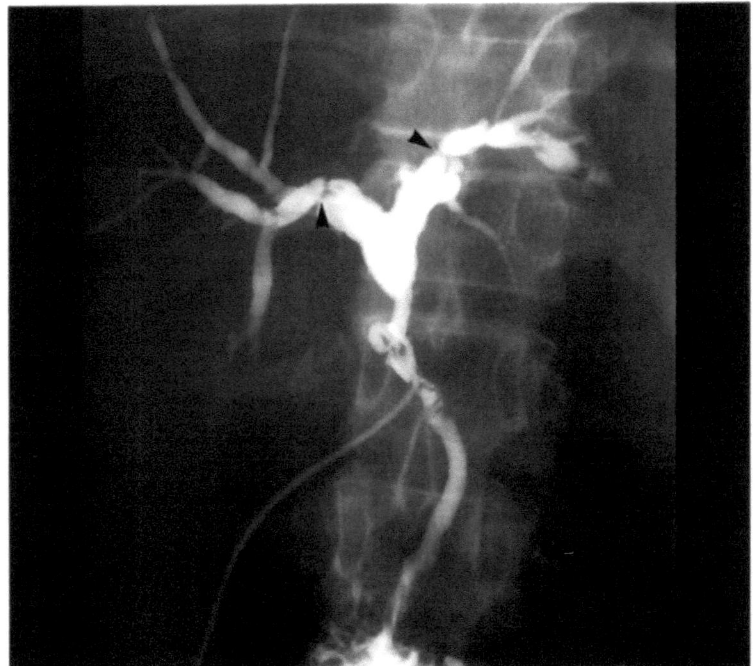

22a

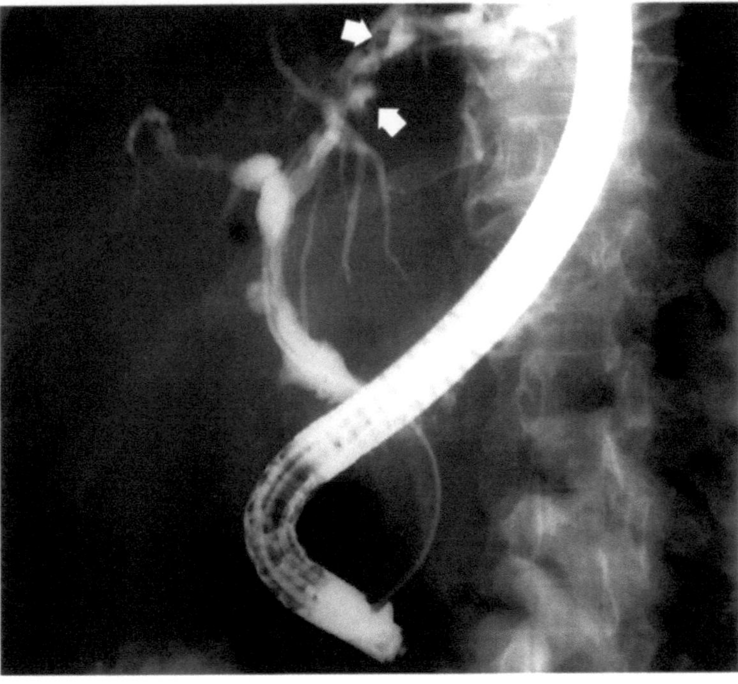

22b

Bile Duct Alterations After Occlusion of the Hepatic Artery

Short Overview

Arterial occlusion following liver transplantation has been reported to occur in 10%–20% [13, 34, 35] of adults and up to 30% [17] of children. The clinical signs of hepatic artery occlusion include fulminant graft failure, persistent graft dysfunction, focal parenchymal necroses, and damage to the biliary tree [35]. The only source of blood supply to the biliary tree is the hepatic artery. Therefore, biliary damage should always be expected to occur following arterial thrombosis. Bile duct damage leads to leakage, biliary strictures, and finally to biliary sepsis [12, 39]. In exceptional cases, hepatic artery occlusion may remain asymptomatic. The radiologic features of ischemic-type lesions resemble those of biliary destruction following arterial thrombosis. Any radiological demonstration of multiple strictures therefore requires angiography. Leaks may occur at the site of anastomosis but also in any other portion of the biliary tree including the intrahepatic ducts. Strictures are numerous, and necrotic material from the ductal wall and debris from superimposed infections form sludge and casts within the biliary system. In those rare cases in which bile duct destruction is limited and restricted mainly to the extrahepatic ducts, surgical repair by a hilar anastomosis may be feasible. This is particularly the case in children. In the overwhelming majority of patients retransplantation is required. For palliation, ischemic biliary lesions may be managed by a percutaneous or endoscopic approach.

Case 23   T-Tube Cholangiogram After Occlusion of the Hepatic Artery

History
A 30-year-old female patient underwent liver transplantation because of acute hepatic failure due to hepatitis B virus infection.

Cholangiography (Fig. 23)

Fig. 23a   The routine T-tube cholangiogram shows a normal postoperative biliary system. There is only rudimentary filling of the left main bile duct. After 6 months the patient experienced acute rejection and was treated with corticosteroids. Transaminases returned to normal, but markers for cholestasis gradually increased. ERC was performed.

Fig. 23b   ERC shows vanishing of the graft's intrahepatic biliary system with multiple small, rounded contrast medium extravasations which must be interpreted as abscesses (*arrows*).

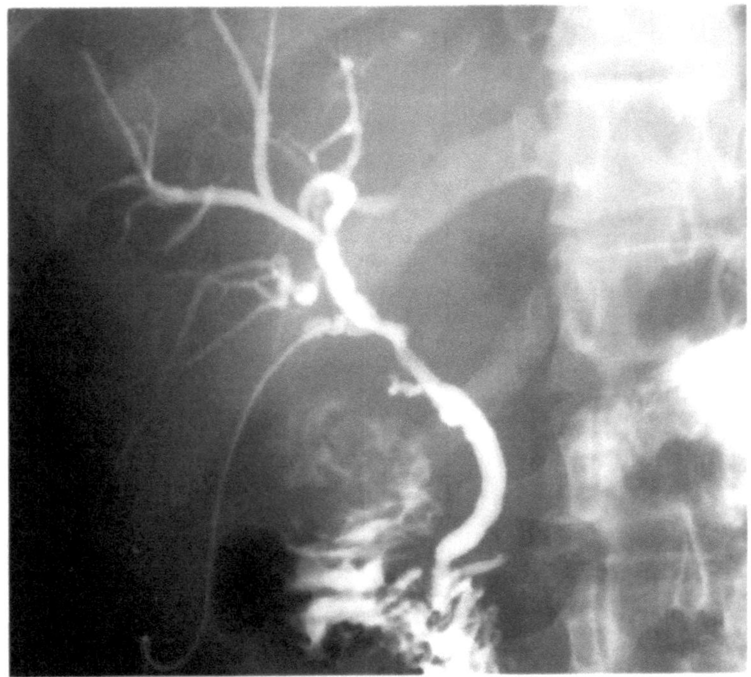

23 a

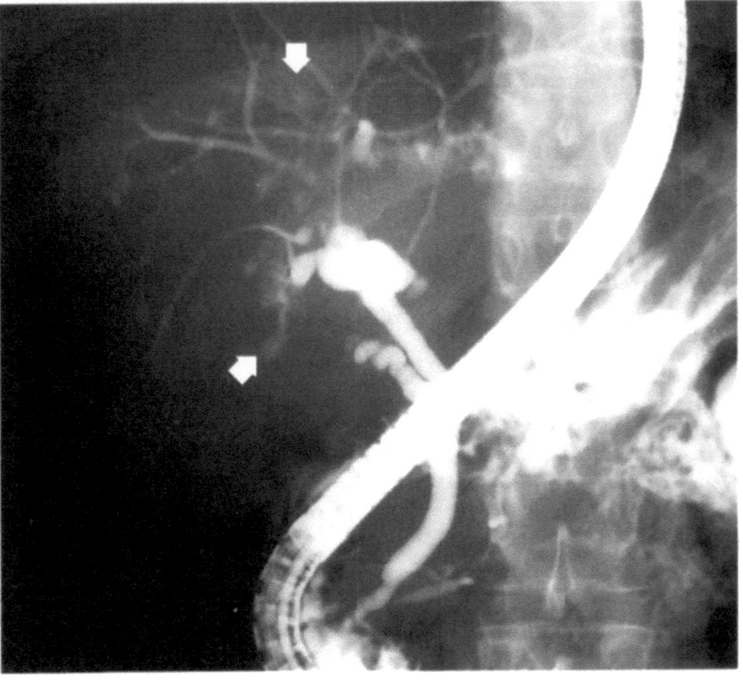

23 b

Fig. 23 c As arterial malperfusion was presumed, an angiogram of the celiac trunk was performed, revealing occlusion of the hepatic artery (*arrow*) and formation of collateral vessels (*arrowheads*). The calibers of the hepatic arteries filled via the collaterals are very small.

Comment

Alteration of the biliary system in this patient was due to occlusion of the hepatic artery which probably occurred during acute rejection of the graft. As collateral vessels are present, occlusion seems to have occurred gradually. The patient underwent retransplantation due to increasing cholestasis and because deterioration of the liver function had started to occur. Examination of the explanted graft showed that all bile ducts were almost completely occluded by sludge.

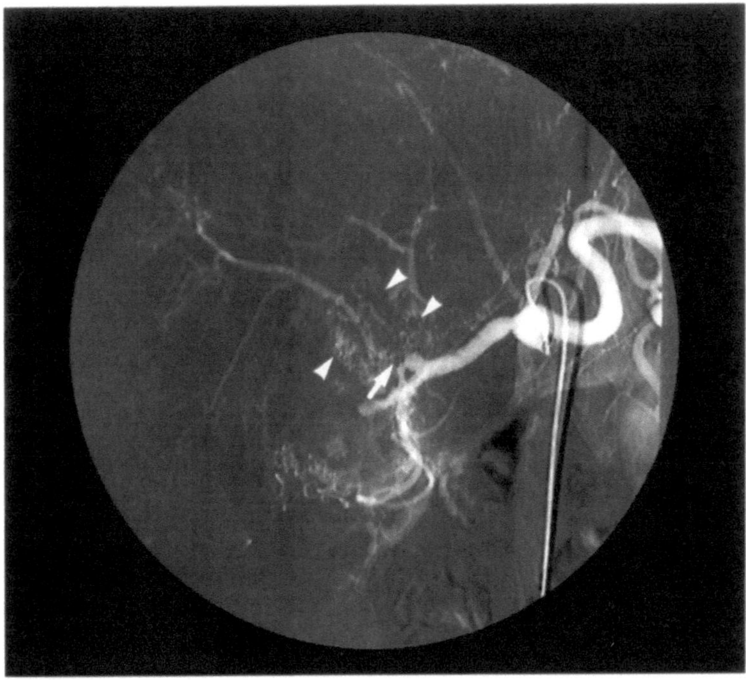

23 c

Case 24 T-Tube Cholangiogram After OLT and Cholangiogram After Occlusion of the Hepatic Artery

History
A 65-year-old female patient underwent liver transplantation because of primary biliary cirrhosis.

Cholangiography (Fig. 24)

Fig. 24 Cholangiography performed via the T-tube 6 weeks after OLT shows several stenoses in segmental and subsegmental branches of the intrahepatic bile ducts (*arrowheads*) and a long high-grade stenosis of the donor's common duct. This must be interpreted as being due to occlusion of the hepatic artery which was demonstrated by celiac angiography. Cold ischemia time had been kept below 10h. Because of deteriorating liver function, the patient underwent retransplantation.

Case 25 Cholangiogram After Occlusion of the Hepatic Artery

History
A 39-year-old female patient underwent liver transplantation because of the Budd-Chiari syndrome. She developed increasing signs of cholestasis 3 months after OLT.

ERC (Fig. 25)

Fig. 25 ERC taken 4 months after OLT showed complete destruction of the extrahepatic biliary system extending into the left duct system with absent filling of the right hepatic system. Arteriography showed occlusion of the hepatic artery as the underlying cause. The patient underwent retransplantation.

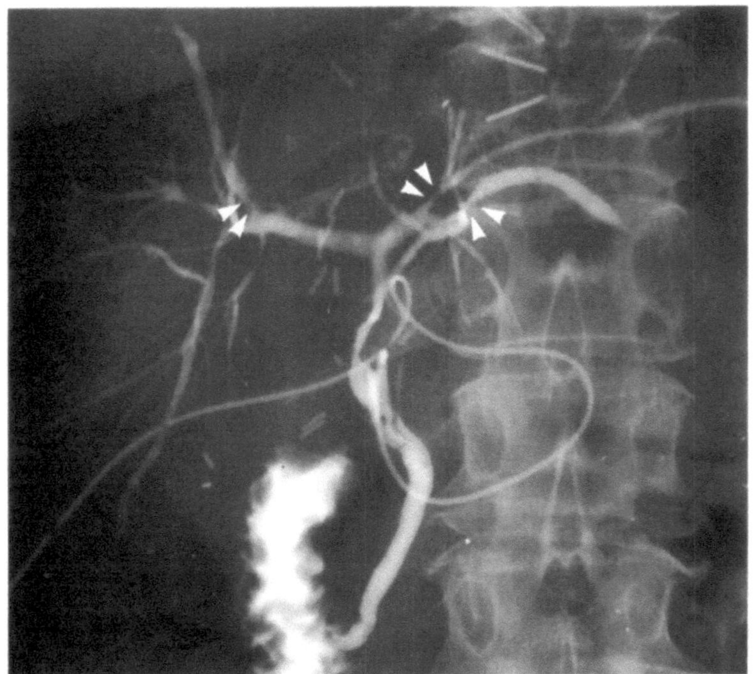

24

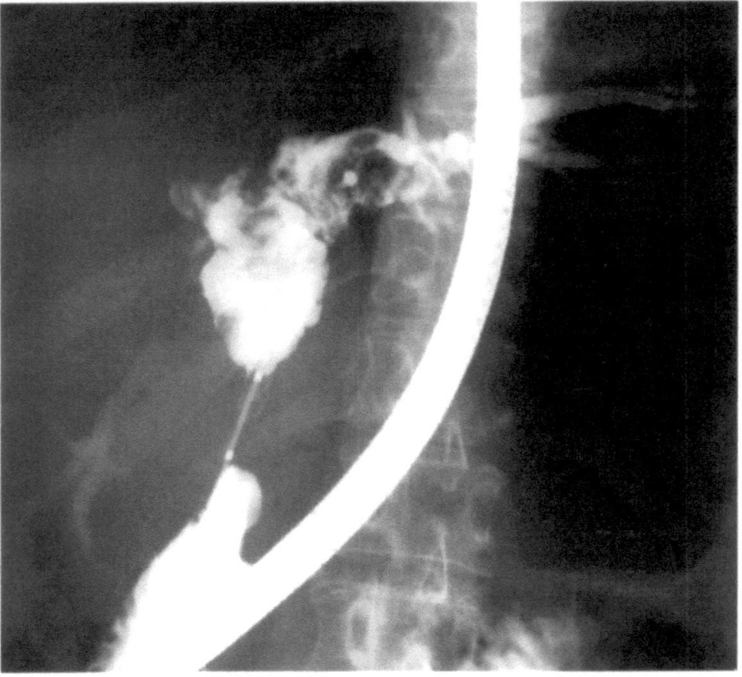

25

Case 26 Cholangiogram After Arterial Malperfusion, Stenosis of the Hepatic Artery, Progression of Bile Duct Alterations, and Percutaneous Treatment; Results of Therapy

History
A 35-year-old female patient underwent liver transplantation because of hemangioendothelioma. After an initial decline with only a slight tendency to normalization, the transaminases remained elevated.

Cholangiography (Fig. 26)

Fig. 26a ERC taken 6 weeks after OLT showed circumscript concentric stenoses (*arrowheads*) and prestenotic dilated intrahepatic ducts.

Fig. 26b Angiography revealed stenosis (*arrows*) and kinking of the hepatic artery. During balloon angioplasty, dissection of the common hepatic artery took place, resulting in deteriorated arterial perfusion which was surgically corrected after a few hours of ischemia.

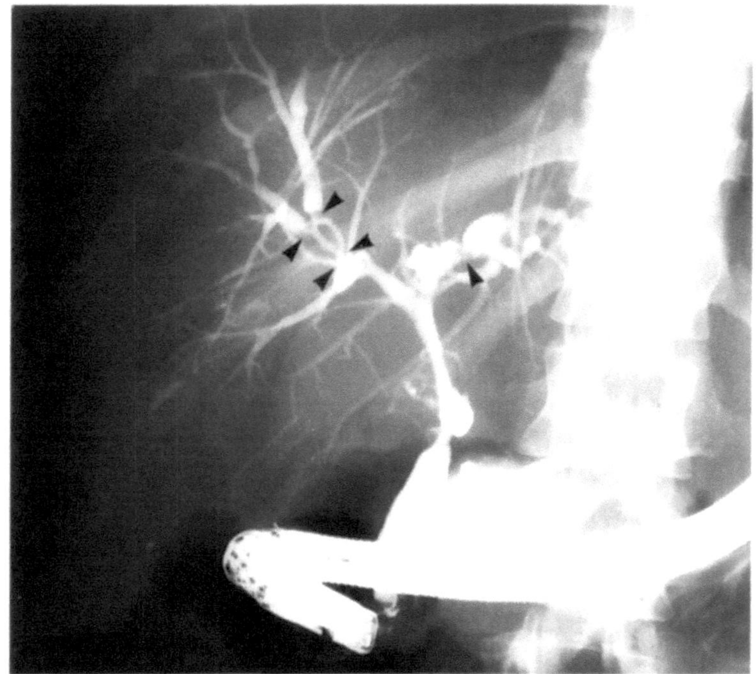

26 a

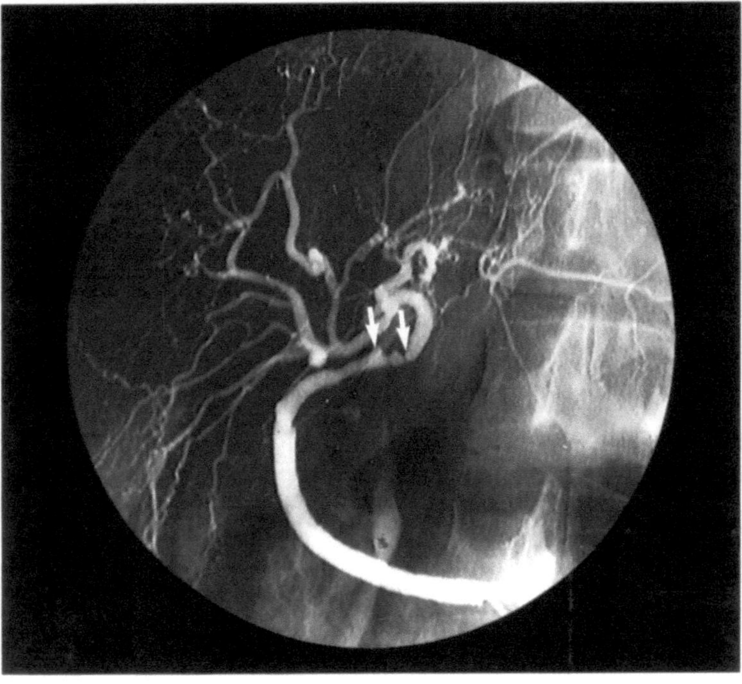

26 b

Fig. 26c ERC taken 10 months after OLT shows rapid progression of bile duct alterations with stenoses, necroses, and sludge in the very poorly outlined intrahepatic bile ducts. Concomitantly, parameters of cholestasis increased.

Fig. 26d The patient underwent percutaneous drainage dilation Duct the biliary system via a lateral and ventral approach, repeated percutanous cholangioscopies, and flushing of the intrahepatic biliary system for a total of 4 months.

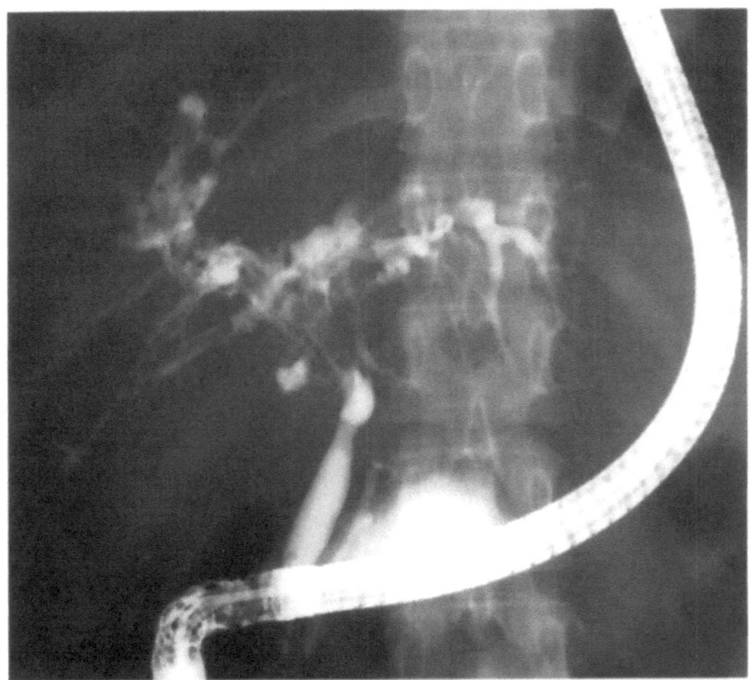

26 c

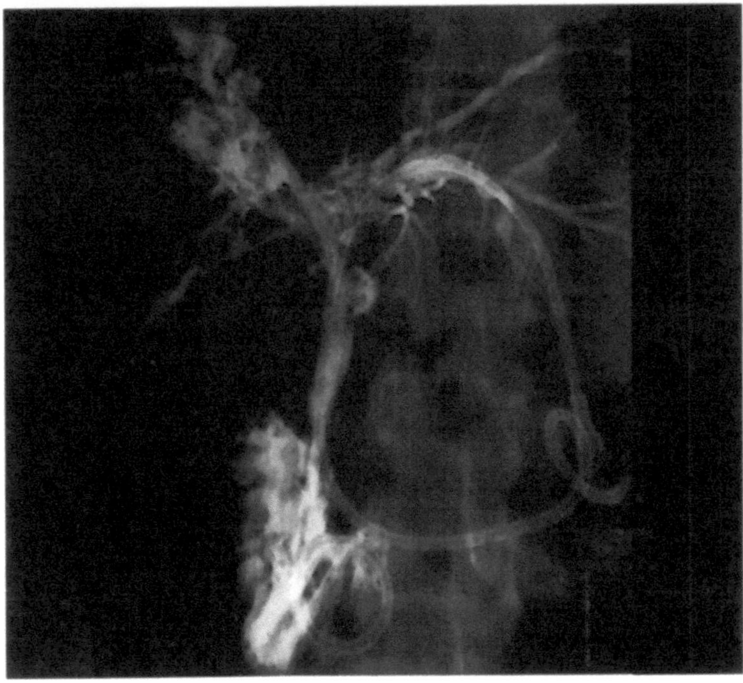

26 d

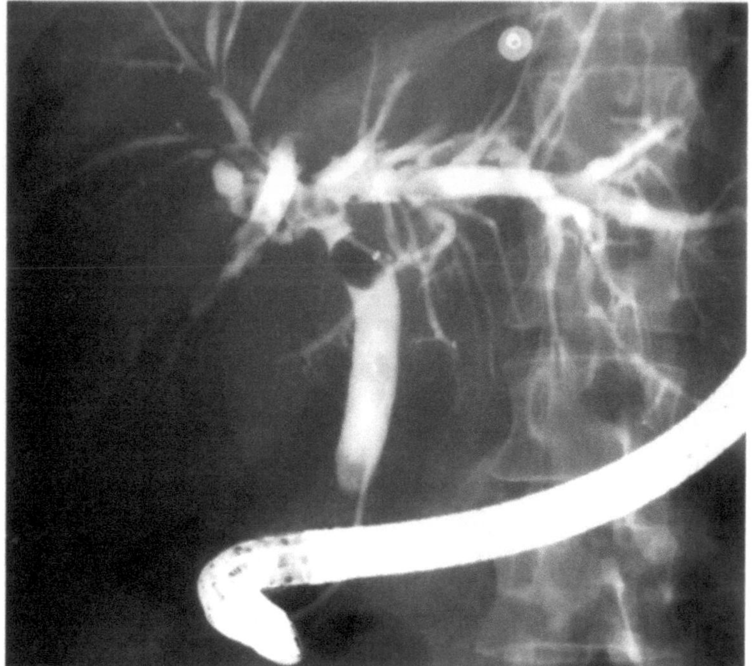

26 e

Fig. 26 e ERC taken 18 months later using a balloon catheter shows that the situation has now considerably improved and consolidated. The patient had normal transaminases and normal cholestasis markers.

Bile Ducts in Chronic Rejection

Short Overview

The pathogenesis of chronic rejection still remains uncertain. Ductopenic or chronic rejection is defined as the absence of interlobular or septal bile ducts from more than 50% of portal tracts, when 20 or more portal tracts are available for histological evaluation [4, 36]. Foam cell arteriopathy is a nonobligatory additional feature of ductopenic rejection. Therefore, two mechanisms may be acting simultaneously or independently of each other in the development of ductopenic rejection. The first is thought to be a direct humoral immunologic insult on the biliary epithelium. The second mechanism is thought to be the result of arterial damage leading to progressive peripheral arterial loss and thereby to a compromised blood supply to the bile ducts. Damage to larger bile ducts is not obligatory for ductopenic rejection and occurs infrequently [3]. The damage to larger ducts accounts for biliary strictures which resemble those following occlusion of the hepatic artery. The frequency of ductopenic rejection after liver transplantation ranges between 2.4% and 20% [16, 22, 36]. Reliable prospective data may be obtained from the large European Multicenter Trial on FK 506 vs cyclosporin A in which ductopenic rejection occurred in 1.4% and 6.4% of cases, respectively [5]. Chronic rejection has been diagnosed between 1 month and 1 year following liver transplantation [36]. The process of chronic rejection has been found to be irreversible with only very few exceptions. Initial reports of the reversibility of chronic rejection with FK 506 treatment could not be confirmed by recent studies [5]. Therefore, retransplantation remains the principal treatment for ductopenic rejection. Unfortunately, up to 90% of patients with ductopenic rejection in the first graft have experienced recurrent ductopenic rejection after retransplantation [36]. Clinical symptoms in chronic rejection are usually caused by damage to the small bile ducts. Therefore, interventional approaches are rarely effective and not advisable.

Case 27 Cholangiogram from a Patient with Chronic Rejection of the Graft

History

A 65-year-old female patient underwent liver transplantation because of primary biliary cirrhosis. She developed histologically proven chronic rejection.

ERC (Fig. 27)

Fig. 27 ERC done 18 months after OLT shows rarefaction of the intrahepatic bile ducts, multiple stenoses, and a generally reduced diameter of the visualized biliary tree.

Comment

Chronic rejection is also described as the "vanishing bile duct syndrome", meaning disappearance of the ducts in the portal triad on light microscopy. Alteration of major ducts may be caused by graft arteriopathy taking place during chronic rejection, as shown in this patient who underwent retransplantation.

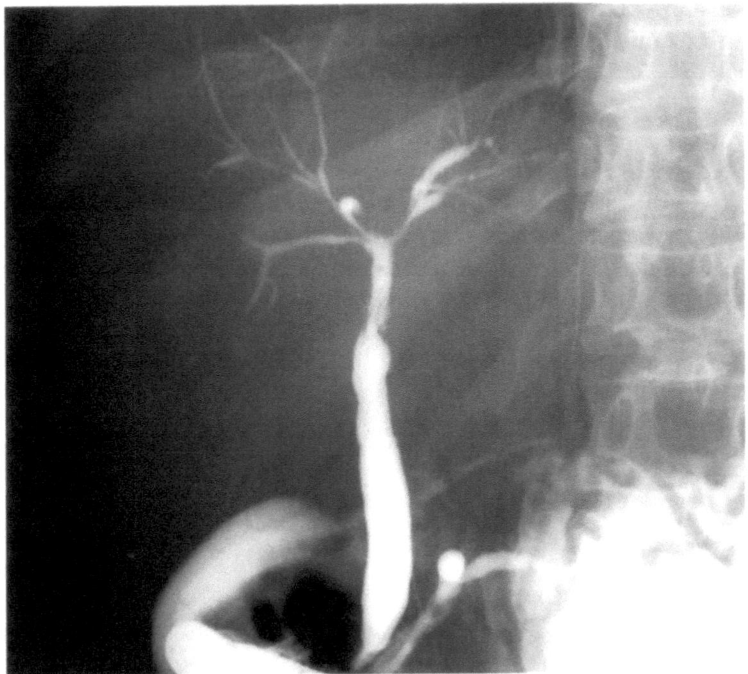

27

Case 28 Initial Alterations of the Hepatic Biliary System in Chronic Rejection; Progression on Follow-Up

History
A 20-year-old male patient underwent liver transplantation because of fulminant hepatic failure induced by hepatitis B virus infection. The patient received an ABO-incompatible graft. He experienced hepatitis B virus reinfection. Four months after OLT, markers of cholestasis increased.

ERC (Fig. 28)

Fig. 28a ERC taken 4 months after transplantation of an ABO-incompatible graft. Diffuse stenoses and early obliteration of the intrahepatic bile ducts are observed (*arrowheads*).

Fig. 28b ERC taken 22 months after OLT reveals partial obstruction and obliteration of the right hepatic duct system (*fat arrows*). Moreover, there is some sludge and the outline of the bifurcation is poorly defined (*arrowheads*).

Comment
As the hepatic artery was patent and the cold ischemia time was less than 10 h, the alterations of the biliary duct system are most probably due to ABO incompatibility resulting in a histological feature comparable to that of chronic rejection. The patients liver funtion deteriorated and retransplantation was necessary.

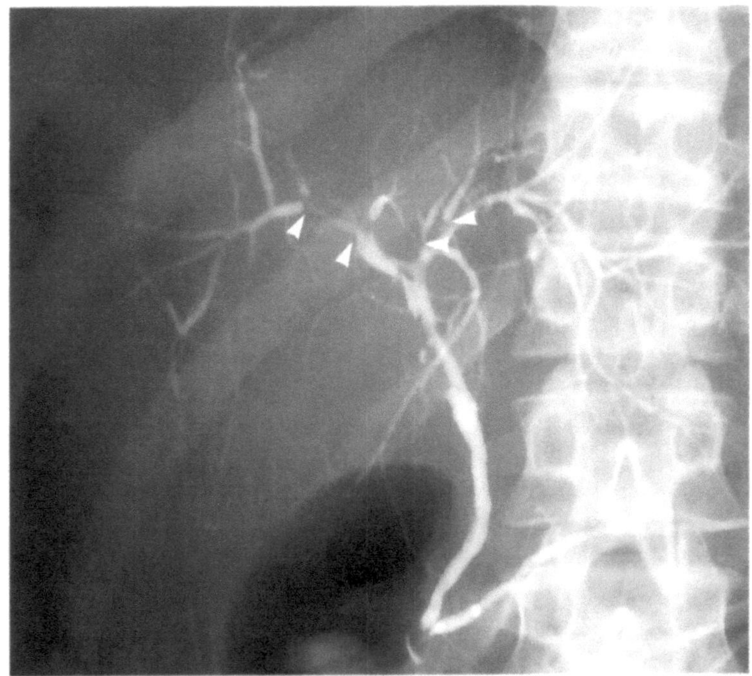

28 a

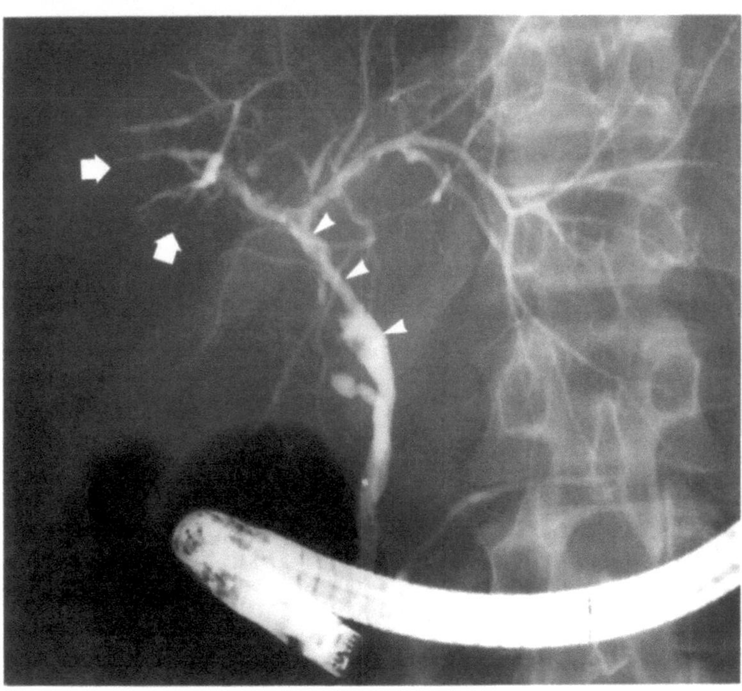

28 b

Case 29 Course of Alterations of the Biliary System in Chronic Rejection

History
A 39-year-old female underwent liver transplantation because of hepatocellular carcinoma. On follow-up studies she developed signs of cholestasis. Liver histology showed chronic rejection.

Cholangiography (Fig. 29)

Fig. 29a Routine T-tube cholangiogram taken 4 weeks after OLT demonstrated a normal biliary system of the graft with concentric stenosis of the anastomosis (*arrowheads*).

Fig. 29b ERC taken 14 months after OLT showed obliteration of most bile ducts.

Comment
Liver histology showed advanced chronic rejection with absence of bile ducts in the periportal fields. The patient did not undergo retransplantation because of tumor recurrence with extrahepatic metastases.

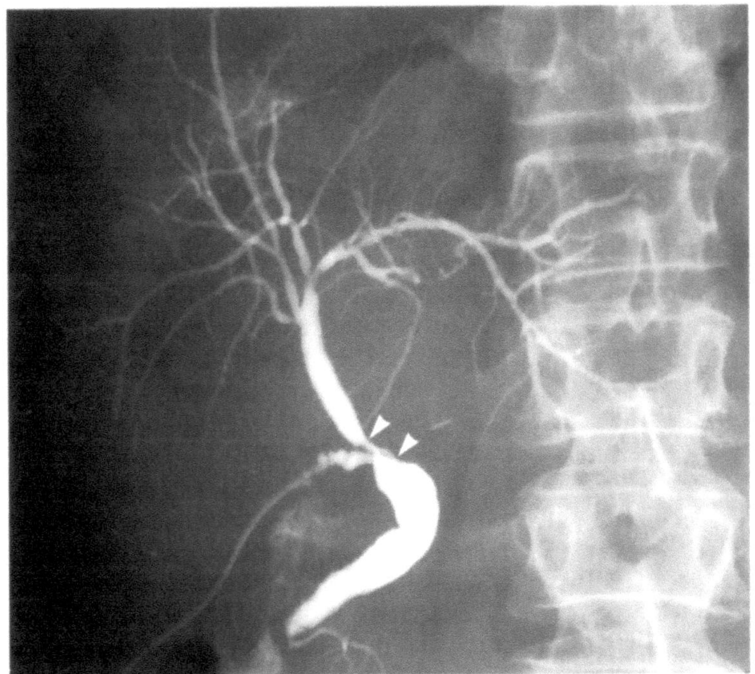

29 a

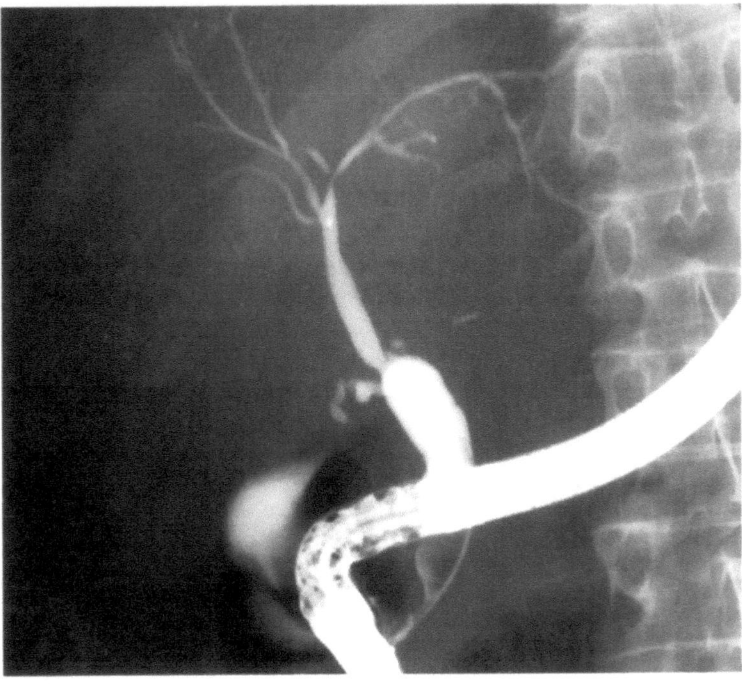

29 b

Disturbed Function of the Sphincter of Oddi

Short Overview

The etiology of this complication is unknown. A possible explanation may be that coordination of the recipient's bile duct motility is permanently disturbed by bile duct dissection and transsection during excision of the diseased liver. The resulting ampullary dysfunction may lead to an increase of alkaline phosphatase and bilirubin. Cholangiographic study reveals the enlarged caliber of both the native and graft duct and a delayed emptying of the contrast material via the papilla. The Pittsburgh group reported 28 patients in whom the bile duct approximately doubled in diameter following transplantation [19]. Ampullary dysfunction is reported to occur in about 2% of the patients [7, 20].

Treatment recommendations differ. In the experience of some authors, endoscopic sphincterotomy proved to be successful [10, 20], while other groups reported treatment failures [7]. The patient's excretory hepatic function failed to normalize and the duct-to-duct anastomosis had to be converted to choledochojejunostomy. Two of our patients experienced this complication and were successfully treated by endoscopic sphincterotomy.

Case 30 Stone in the Recipient's Dilated Common Bile Duct

History

A 55-year-old male patient underwent liver transplantation because of alcohol-induced liver cirrhosis. He developed signs of cholestasis 26 months after OLT.

ERC (Fig. 30)

Fig. 30 ERC at 26 months after OLT revealed a large radiolucent distal common bile duct stone below the site of anastomosis (*arrows*). Endoscopic sphincterotomy was performed. Extraction was not possible. Therefore the stone was fragmented by extracorporal lithotripsy and the remnants were removed with Dormia baskets and balloon extractors. Chemical analysis revealed a bilirubin concrement.

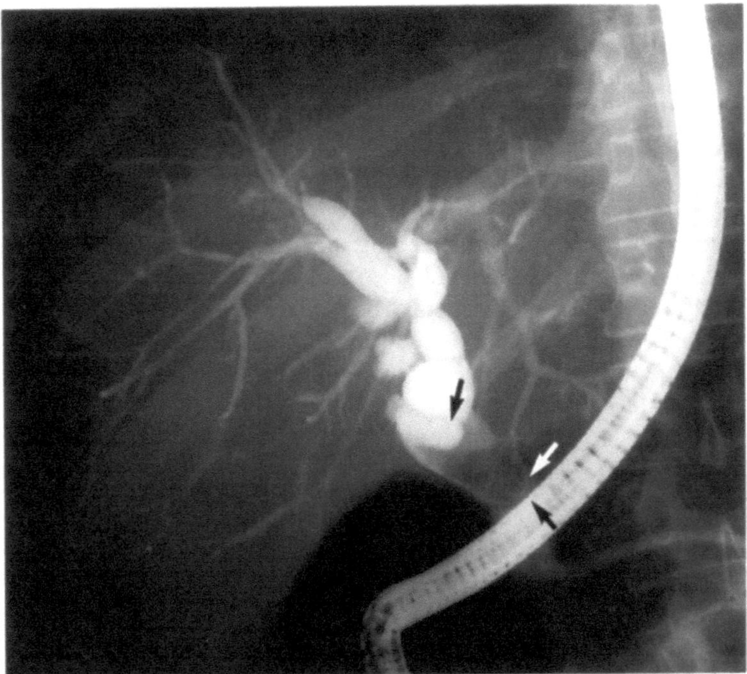

30

Comment

OLT frequently results in functional disturbances of the sphincter of Oddi. This is probably due to damage to the innervation of the sphincter caused by the transplantation procedure. Bile stasis and subsequent formation of gallstones may occur.

Case 31 Dilated Common Duct in the Recipient and Stenoses of the Main Hepatic Ducts

History

A 27-year-old male patient underwent liver transplantation because of hepatitis B virus-induced cirrhosis. One year after transplantation diffuse bleeding occurred in the duodenum. Embolization by placement of a minicoil was unsuccessful and laparatomy was performed. The source of bleeding was two small arteries in the postpyloric duodenum without any evidence of ulceration. The arteries were oversewn. After 3 years the patient developed signs of cholestasis.

ERC (Fig. 31)

Fig. 31 a ERC shows excessive dilation of the recipient's choledochal duct. A balloon catheter was inflated to deliver sufficient contrast medium to visualize the proximal biliary system. Circumscript stenoses of the bile duct bifurcation are present (*arrows*).

Fig. 31 b Endoscopic sphicterotomy was performed. A stenosis of the right hepatic duct was passed with a guide wire and a rigid 5F dilatator was then advanced. Dilation was subsequently performed. Stenosis of the left duct was treated the same way.

Comment

Enlargement of the recipient's common bile duct is probably due to a disturbed function of the sphincter of Oddi. This may have been a consequence of the previous relaparatomy to stop duodenal bleeding. The reason for the stenoses of both bile ducts occurring late after transplantation remains unclear.

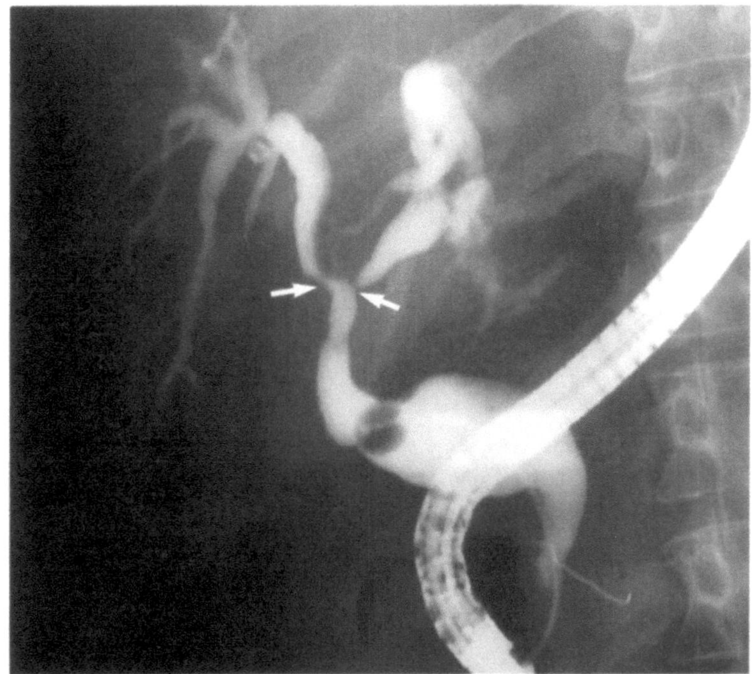

31 a

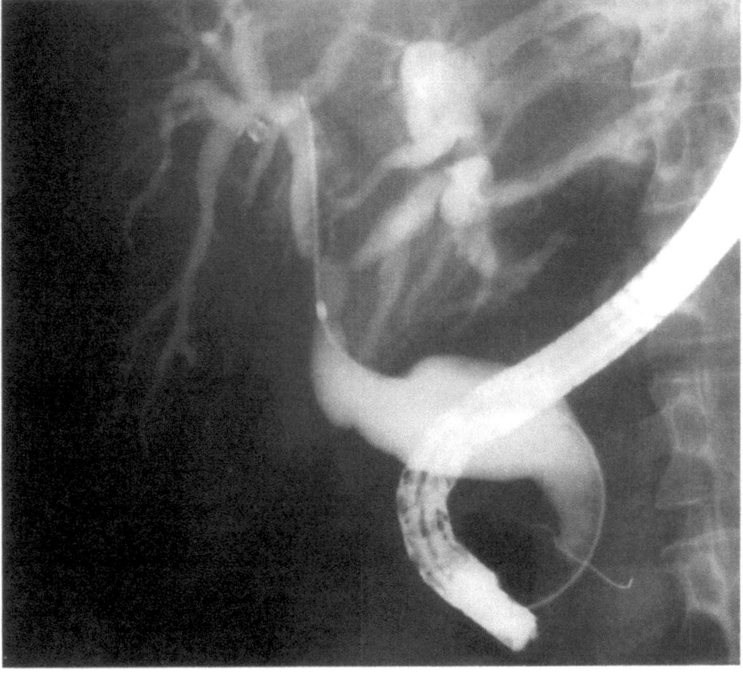

31 b

References

1. Chaib E, Friend PJ, Jamieson NV, Calne RY (1994) Biliary tract reconstruction: comparison of different techniques after 187 paediatric liver transplantations. Transpl Int 7:39–42
2. Colonna JO, Shaked A, Gomes AS, Colquhoun SD, et al (1992) Biliary strictures complicating liver transplantation. Incidence, pathogenesis, management and outcome. Ann Surg 216: 344–350
3. Demetris AJ, Jaffe R, Starzl TE (1987) A review of adult and pediatric post-transplant liver pathology. Pathol Annu (Part II): 347–386
4. Demetris AJ, Shiquang Q, Hong S, Fung JJ (1990) Liver allograft rejection: an overview of morphologic findings. Am J Surg Pathol 14:49–63
5. European FK 506 Multicentre Liver Study Group (1994) Randomised trial comparing tacrolimus (FK 506) and cyclosporin in prevention of liver allograft rejection. The Lancet 344:423–428
6. Golling M, Datsis K, Ioannidis P, v Frankenberg M, et al (1995) Einfluß der Anastomosenrekonstruktion auf vaskuläre Komplikationen nach Lebertransplantation. Zentralbl Chir 120:445–449
7. Greif F, Bronsther, OL, Van Thiel DH, Casavilla A, et al (1994) The incidence, timing and management of biliary tract complications after orthotopic liver transplantation. Ann Surg 219:40–45
8. Iwatsuki SI, Shaw BW Jr, Starzl TE (1983) Biliary tract complications in liver transplantation under cyclosporine-steroid therapy. Transplant Proc 15:1288
9. Kadmon M, Bleyl JU, Küppers B, Otto G, Herfarth Ch (1993) Biliary complications after prolonged UW preservation of liver allografts. Transplant Proc 25:1651–1652
10. LaBerge JM, Ostroff JW (1993) Nonoperative management of biliary tract complications after liver transplantation. Sem Gastrointest Dis 4:170–177
11. Lallier M, St Vil D, Luks FI, LaBerge JM, et al (1993) Biliary tract complications in pediatric orthotopic liver transplantation. J Pediatr Surg 28:1102–1105
12. Langnas AN, Marujo W, Stratta RJ, Wood RP, et al (1991) Vascular complications after orthotopic liver transplantation. Am J Surg 161:76–82
13. Lebeau G, Yanaga K, Marsh JW, Tzakis AG et al (1990) Analysis of surgical complications after 397 hepatic transplantations. Surg Gynecol Obstet 170:317–322
14. Lerut J, Gordon RD, Iwatsuki S, Esquivel CO, et al (1987) Biliary tract complications in human orthotopic liver transplantation. Transplantation 43:47–51

15. Li S, Stratta RJ, Langnas AN, Wood RP, et al (1992) Diffuse biliary tract injury after orthotopic liver transplantation. Am J Surg 164:536–540

16. Ludwig J, Wiesner RH, Batts KP, Perkins JD, Krom RAF (1987) Acute vanishing bile duct syndrome (acute irreversible rejection) after orthotopic liver transplantation. Hepatology 7:476–483

17. Mazzaferro V, Esquivel CO, Makowka L, Belle S, et al (1989) Hepatic artery thrombosis after pediatric liver transplantation: Medical or surgical event? Transplantation 47:971–977

18. McMaster P, Herbertson BM, Cusick C, Calne RY, et al (1979) The developement of biliary "sludge" following liver transplantation. Transpl Proc 11:262–266

19. Miller WJ, Campbell WL, Zajko AB, Pinna A, et al (1991) Obstructive dilatation of extrahepatic recipient and donor bile ducts complicating orthotopic liver transplantation: imaging and laboratory findings. Am J Roentgenol 157:29–32

20. Neuhaus P, Blumhardt G, Bechstein WO, Steffen R, et al (1994) Technique and results of biliary reconstruction using side-to-side choledochocholedochostomy in 300 orthotopic liver transplantations. Ann Surg 219:426–434

21. Neuhaus P, Brölsch C, Ringe B, Lauchart W, et al (1984) Results of biliary reconstruction after liver transplantation. Transpl Proc 16:1225–1227

22. Oguma S, Belle S, Starzl TE, Demetris AJ (1989) A histometric analysis of chronically rejected human liver allografts: insights into the mechanisms of bile duct loss: direct immunologic and ischemic factors. Hepatol 9:204–209

23. Otto G, Roeren T, Golling M, Datsis K et al. (1995) Ischemic type lesions der Gallenwege nach Lebertransplantation: 2-Jahres-Ergebnisse. Zentralbl Chir 120:450–454

24. Rath AM, Zhang J, Bourdelat D, Chevrel JP (1993) Arterial vascularisation of the extrahepatic biliary tract. Surg Radiol Anat 15:105–111

25. Rouch DA, Emond JC, Thistlethwaite JR Jr, Mayes JT, Broelsch CE (1990) Choledochocholedochostomy without a T-tube or internal stent in transplantation of the liver. Surg Gynecol Obstet 170:239–244

26. Sanchez-Urdazpal L, Gores GJ, Ward E, Maus TP, et al (1992) Ischemic type biliary complications after orthotopic liver transplantation. Hepatology 16: 49–53

27. Sanchez-Urdazpal L, Gores GJ, Ward EM, Maus TP, et al (1993) Diagnostic features and clinical outcome of ischemic type biliary complications after liver transplantation. Hepatology 17: 605–609

28. Saxena R, Tokat Y, Soin AS, Rasmussen A, et al (1995) Relationship between patterns of hepatobiliary vascular supply and biliary complications in liver transplantation: An anatomical and clinical analysis. Transplant Proc 27:1199–1200

29. Senninger N, Datsis K, Ioannidis P, v Frankenberg M, et al (in press) „Gallengangsrekonstruktion bei Lebertransplantation – Komplikationen und Reeingriffe". Zentralbl Chir

30. Sheng R, Sammon JK, Zajko AB, Campbell WL (1994) Bile leak after hepatic transplantation: cholangiographic features, prevalence and clinical outcome. Radiology 192:413–416
31. Stratta RJ, Wood RP, Langnas AN, Hollins RR, et al (1989) Diagnosis and treatment of biliary complications after orthotopic liver transplantation. Surgery 106:675–683
32. Terblanche J, Allison HF, Northover JMA (1982) An ischemic basis for biliary strictures. Surgery 94:52–57
33. Theilmann L, Küppers B, Kadmon M, Roeren T, et al (1994) Biliary tract strictures after orthotopic liver transplantation: diagnosis and management. Endoscopy 26:517–522
34. Todo S, Makowka L, Tzakis AG, Marsch JW, et al (1987) Hepatic artery in liver transplantation. Transplant Proc 19:2406–2411
35. Tzakis AG, Gordon RD, Shaw BW Jr, Iwatsuki S, Starzl TE (1985) Clinical presentation of hepatic artery thrombosis after liver transplantation in the cyclosporine era. Transplantation 40:667–671
36. Van Hoek B, Wiesner RH, Krom RAF, Ludwig J Moore SB (1992) Severe ductopenic rejection following liver transplantation: Incidence, time of onset, risk factors, treatment and outcome. Sem Liver Dis 12:41–50
37. Ward EM, Kiely MJ, Maus TP, et al (1990) Hilar biliary strictures after liver transplantation: Cholangiography and percutaneous treatment. Radiology 177:259–263
38. Zajko AB, Campbell WL, Bron KM, Lecky JW, et al (1985) Cholangiography and interventional biliary radiology in adult liver transplantation. Am J Roentgenol 44: 127–133
39. Zajko AB, Campbell WL, Logsdon GA, Bron KM, et al (1987) Cholangiographic findings in hepatic artery occlusion after liver transplantation. Am J Roentgenol 149:485–489
40. Zemel G, Zajko AB, Skolnick ML, Bron KM, Campbell WL (1988) The role of sonography and transhepatic cholangiography in the diagnosis of biliary complications after liver transplantation. Am J Roentgenol 151:943–946